Ayurveda

– in Everyday Life

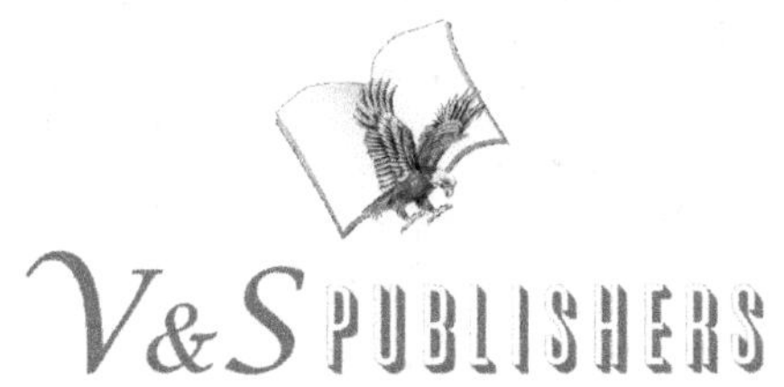

V&S PUBLISHERS

Published by

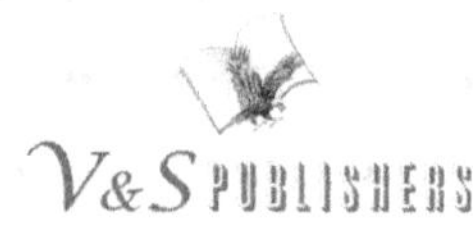

V&S PUBLISHERS

F-2/16, Ansari Road, Daryaganj, New Delhi-110002
☎ 011-23240026, 011-23240027 • *Fax* 011-23240028
Email info@vspublishers.com • *Website* www.vspublishers.com

Regional Office Hyderabad

5-1-707/1, Brij Bhawan (Beside Central Bank of India Lane)
Bank Street, Koti, Hyderabad - 500 095
☎ 040-24737290
E-mail vspublishershyd@gmail.com

Branch Office : Mumbai

Jaywant Industrial Estate, 1st Floor-108, Tardeo Road
Opposite Sobo Central, Mumbai - 400 034
☎ 022-23510736
E-mail: vspublishersmum@gmail.com

BUY OUR BOOKS FROM: AMAZON FLIPKART

© Copyright V&S PUBLISHERS
ISBN 978-93-579414-6-4

Edition 2020

Publisher's Note

Continuing with our 'Alternative Therapy health Series', we now discuss the uses and benefits derived from Aromatherapy. Aromatherapy has been around for more than 6000 years. In this form of complementary and supplementary therapy, it is the aroma oils that offer miraculous properties to heal and cure our overall well-being. Essential oils are one of the world's great untapped resources. This complete volume explains how to incorporate these ancient medicines into everyday life for personal care, physical and mental health, and a safe home environment. It explains the properties, uses and benefits derived from 57 essential oils as alternatives to often toxic human-made health, beauty, and cleaning products.

Laying to rest old arguments over essential oils' alleged toxicity and whether they can be ingested or used undiluted, this book presents simple recipes and protocols for treating and preventing common ailments, such as colds, flu, herpes, and candida, as well as for pain management. Offering new essential oil treatment opportunities for hepatitis, osteoporosis, liver detoxification, and the prevention of UV damage and melanoma, the author shows how essential oils can also ameliorate the debilitating side effects of chemotherapy and other cancer treatments as well as how even home use of essential oils for relaxation or skin care can help build one's immunity and overall well-being.

Kindly treat the below mentioned as a Disclaimer of sorts :

The Editorial Board writes in this book their opinion and that there may be many people who disagree with the conclusions. The publisher and the author, the distributors and bookstores, present this information for educational purposes only. This book is not making an attempt to prescribe any medical treatment; the knowledge given is just passing the acquired experience.

This book is only composed of opinions and conclusions of Editorial Board. The readers are requested to seek medical advice before blindly following the book. The Publisher/Authors shall not be liable for consequences thereafter.

Preface

This book grew out to meet the burgeoning need for more professional knowledge about non-mainstream approaches in physical and mental well being. This need to spread awareness has been fueled by the huge consumer-driven trend toward these treatments over the last 2-3 decades. This text aims to provide a reader with cutting edge information from many diverse areas of alternative, complementary, and innovative clinical practice in the area of physical well being and emotional health. The purpose of this work is threefold:

1. To offer a broader, deeper view of information from areas that, although outside mainstream practice, are having an increasing impact and demand.
2. To offer a sense of the level of scientific research and experience associated with complementary and supplementary fields in the area of total health.
3. To further explore and incorporate new treatment options. This text, while not exhaustive, provides a fair overview from the cutting edge of change in health care practices. The overall layout of this 'Alternative Health Care Series' demonstrates the body-mind-spirit premise that permeates diverse field of treatment. By its very nature, this type of book is more focused on divisions and separations-- different topics, different sections, and different treatments. Each section begins with a description of the treatment, its safety and/or contraindications, scientific documentation of its efficacy, discussion of which ailment it is best used for, and other important references. Time has come for

physicians, clinicians and therapists to have a look at how the marriage of conventional health care to complementary and alternative therapies can offer improved diagnosis than either can alone. The text will offer them more knowledge, a broader viewpoint, and greater option to practice and care for those under their care and attention.

Table of Content's

ABC of Ayurveda

Ayurveda is an ancient medicine system of the Indian subcontinent. The word Ayurveda has been a conjugation of two Sanskrit words ayus, meaning 'life' and veda, meaning 'science', thus ayurveda literally means the 'science of life'. Unlike other traditional medicinal systems, Ayurveda is more focused on simple and logical therapies. It is in fact a set of practical and simple guidelines for long life and good health. The basic feature of this medicinal therapy is the internal harmony of various body parts as well as body's harmony with the surrounding nature and environment. Ayurveda in contemporary times is recognized by the western world to be a form of complementary and alternative medicine.

The Origin

The existence of Ayurvedic medicinal therapy can be traced back to the origins of Vedas- Atharveda in particular. It is said that the Sushruta Samhita, the main text book of Ayurvedic medicine system written by famous Vaidya Sushruta appeared during the 1st millennium BCE. The other famous book for Ayurvedic studies is 'Charak Samhita', the one written by another famous Vaidya of ancient India, Charak. It is said that in ancient era, Ayurveda was one of the most advance medicinal therapies with the prescribed treatment for complex ailments like angina pectoris, diabetes, hypertension, stones as well as surgeries like plastic surgery, cataract surgery and anal fistulas.

The Branches

Unlike other traditional medicinal therapies, Ayurveda believes in specialized treatment. It branches itself into eight different categories to deal with eight different kinds of ailments. The Kaaya Cikitsaa, Baala Cikitsaa, Graha Chikitsa, S`aalakya Tantra, Agada Tantra, Rasayan Tantra, Vajeekarana Cikitsaa and the S`alya Tantra are the eight different branches of Ayurveda dealing with internal medicine, pediatrics, psychiatry, treatment of head and neck, toxicology, rejuvenation therapy, reproductive medicines and surgery.

Practical Guidelines

Other than mere treatment of ailments, Ayurveda also suggests practical guidelines for living healthy. It asks for striking balance between three substances: wind/spirit/air, phlegm, and bile, each representing divine forces necessary for a healthy body, mind or soul. Ayurveda also suggests consumption of right kind of diet. The suggestions for diet in Ayurvedic texts range from preparation and consumption of food, to healthy routines for day and night, sexual life, and rules for ethical conduct.

Ayurveda stresses on moderation in food intake, sleep, sexual intercourse and the intake of medicine. Most of the time, Ayurveda suggests the use of vegetable drugs; however the use of animal product and minerals in the Ayurvedic treatment are also not uncommon. Hundreds of vegetable drugs like cardamom and cinnamon are used in the treatment of various kinds of ailments. Animal products like milk, bones and gallstones and minerals like sulphur, arsenic, lead, copper sulphate and gold are also used in Ayurvedic medicines.

There are many advantages to using Ayurvedic remedies. They can be used to treat and prevent illnesses and diseases. Ayurvedic remedies are formulated using herbs that cause little or no side effects. Besides their healing properties, the herbs used in Ayurvedic medicine also relax the body and mind, promote balance and ensure efficient functioning.

Ayurvedic remedies are available in various forms including: fresh juices made from herbs; Churna (herbs that have been powdered and taken with food or water for internal and external uses); Ghrat (herbs cooked in clarified butter or ghee); Arka (a distillate made from herbs); Quath (crushed or ground herbs that are used as a brew or a decoction); Anjan or Dhoop (liniments, drops or paste that are usually applied externally); Modak or Paak (herbs that have been cooked in sugar or jaggery); and Asav or Arista (a light wine made through the fermentation of herbs).

History of Ayurveda

Ayurveda is a traditional holistic health care system that has been practiced in India for more than 5000 years. With its origin deeply seated in the hinterlands of India ayurveda is an elaborated medical system and is regarded as the oldest form of health care in the world. Ayurveda is a Sanskrit term, made up of the words "ayus" and "veda." "Ayus" means life and "Veda" means knowledge or science. The term "ayurveda" thus means the knowledge of life or the science of life. According to the ancient Ayurvedic scholar Charaka, "ayu" comprises the mind, body, senses and the soul. It analyses the human body in terms of earth, water, fire, air and ether as well as the three bodily humors.

In India the origin of ayurveda is as old as the religion, Hinduism. There were originally four main books of spirituality, which included among other topics, health, astrology, spiritual business, government, army, poetry and behaviour. These books are known as the four Vedas like the Rig Veda, Sama Veda, Yajur Veda and Atharva Veda. Ayurveda was a sub section attached to the Atharva Veda and is treated as Upaveda of Rigveda and Antharveda (internal part) of Atharvana veda.

Myths and legends lace the origin of this traditional health care system. It is believed that ayurveda was once communicated to the Indian saints and sages. Myths unfold that Dhanvanatri, the physician of the gods in Hindu mythology, penned down ayurveda and taught it to the sages.

While according to another legend, the knowledge of healing, ayurveda originated from Lord Brahma who taught it to Daksha, who further taught it to Lord Indra. There is an interesting story which indicates the origin and development of ayurveda as a holistic treatment in India. It was the time of sheer restlessness; Human existence was under the lash of deaths and disease and it was then to offer human being a solution the great sages gathered together. During this meeting, saint Bharadvaja came forward and learnt the science of ayurveda from Indra. Bharadvaja then taught ayurveda to Atreya who further carried ayurveda as a treatment procedure to the next level of maturity and transmitted this knowledge throughout world. Later it was Agnivesha, the disciples of Atreya who wrote Agnivesha Samhita which is still considered as the most comprehensive form of Ayurveda. However, in later days the classical texts, Charaka Samhita (Charaka), Ashtanga Hridaya (Vagbhata) and Susruta Samhita (Susruta) formed the foundation of ayurveda.

Ayurveda, as a holistic treatment procedure thus represents the science of life and longevity originating in the Vedic traditions of India. Based on the principle of eternal life, ayurveda has a vast body of knowledge which covers eight principal branches. The primary element of ayurveda involves the eternal symbiosis of mind, body and spirit for a healthy living. Any imbalance in this symbiosis of body, spirit and mind indeed results in physical ailments. Ayurveda as a treatment concept thus re-establishes the harmony between the body and its habitat by creating the optimum health environment.

The whole science of ayurveda is based on the `Five Great Elements` known as Panchabhuta theory. These five elements are earth (prithvi), water (jal), fire (agni or tej), air (vayu) and ether or space (akash). In ayurvedic tradition the universe is made up of these five elements. According to ayurveda therefore the origin of all aspects of existence is consciousness. Matter and Energy are one; however, matter is manifested in the Panchabhuta or the five elements. Ayurveda also perceives the body, the mind and the spirit likewise and therefore zero down specific methods for working on each to ensure healthy living.

Ayurveda recognizes three main energies that combine to form all things in the universe. These are recognized as being fundamental to all life and are seen in the processes of growth, maintenance, and decay. Their actions are named anabolism, metabolism, and catabolism in the western sciences. Life, light, and love represent all these energies and are found in the environments at almost every moment and on every level. When people become aware of these qualities within themselves, they take the first steps toward creating a healthy life. Ayurveda assists in identifying these energies in a person's body and shows them how to more fully experience these gifts and gain freedom from their limitations. By working with the body's unique nature, true health can be created. Ayurveda names these basic energies as Vata (ether/air), Pitta (fire) and Kapha (water/earth). Vata rules mental mobility. Pitta, or fire, governs digestion and assimilation on all levels from food to ideas. Kapha or water rules the form and substance and is responsible for weight, cohesion and stability. In the Ayurvedic approach to life and health, it is recognized how these energies work at each moment in people's bodies and minds. When these energies are recognized, countering the destructive forces with positive actions becomes possible. This further creates balance.

Ayurveda insists that any discordant note in the synthesis of the spirit, body and mind due to external or internal causes is a cause for concern. The `fault` or dosha, the `tissue` or dhatu and the `impurity` or mala should be in perfect harmony with each other, with all the components properly balanced and that is the secret of health as per ayurveda. Quite ideally therefore the treatment in ayurveda also concentrates on the symbiosis of the spirit, mind and the body. Essentially ayurveda holds the view that it is the tridosha imbalance, which causes illness. Other causes are the imbalance of digestive fire (agni), and accumulation of toxins (ama) formed by undigested nutrients and psychological experiences. The therapeutic measures in ayurveda are therefore taken both to prevent diseases and also to cure them. Thus ayurvedic procedures are done either to detoxify the body or as a prelude to strengthening the immune system. Panchakarma or `five procedures`, is the most sought after detoxification therapy in ayurveda which paves the way for the culmination of ayurvedic treatment of healing whilst ensuring health.

The legacy of ayurveda as a treatment method which was initiated by the early ayurvedic practitioners like the Shusruta, Charaka or Vagbhata is still regarded as one of the reigning alternative treatment methods in India. With the promise of the profound expression of the holistic nature of good health, ayurveda as a holistic healing method has been perfected over ages. Just not the cure from disease ayurveda is the science of life which views a healthy individual as an integral synthesis of mind, body and spirit, living in harmony with fellow beings and environment.

Principles of Ayurveda

Ayurveda is not a medicinal approach to the issue of health rather this ancient science is defined as the complete philosophy of life. Ayurveda gives full importance to each and every aspect of life and is well reckoned as one of the most well accepted holistic treatment procedure with a rich tradition of more than five thousand years. It is a view of life and it absolutely understands the non-material components of human life that are the thoughts, consciousness and thoughts. There are several aspects of this traditional system of medicine, which discriminates it from other approaches to health care. The principle of Ayurveda is based on the 'Five Great Elements' termed as the Panchabhuta theory. These five elements are Earth (prithvi), Water (jal), Fire (agni), Air (vayu) and Space (akash). The principle of Ayurveda perceives body, mind and spirit.

Ayurveda defines that the four basic aspects of life - 'atma' (the soul), 'manas' (the mind), 'indriyas' (the senses) and 'sharira' (the body) have their specific functions and that contribute to the completeness of life. Ayurveda mainly focuses on a balanced and integrated relationship among these four components. It also focuses on establishing and maintaining balance of the life energies within the individual rather than focusing on individual symptoms. The principle of Ayurveda is based on the self healing process where the individual's inherent tendency is to move from the diseased state towards the healthy state. In order to have a full knowledge and understanding of the functions of the body, understanding the senses of the body is very essential.

Atma: The Soul

Atma is defined as the motivating intelligence that guides the human mind and life. Though, it is also said that atma is actually the least tangible part of human life. This is more clearly defined as the 'sense of I' and is the source of unseen guiding force. Each and every aspect of life has inherent coordination with other parts of the body. The principle of atma is also defined as the governing principle that existed within as a part of human beings. Further, this guiding principle has two aspects, first one being the 'jiva atma'. In the case of first one, intelligence is associated with entire concept of 'soul'. It guides as per the particular destiny of an individual's life. The second aspect is the 'param atma' or more commonly defined as the universal soul. It is the very consciousness of the nature and it is the essence of the individual soul. 'Param atma' is responsible for unifying all diversity of nature. In short, 'jiva atma' is an appearance of the 'param atma'.

Manas: The Mind

Ayurveda specifies that all the happiness or unhappiness, health or ill-health and all the feelings arise in human mind first. Soul or atma is defined as the director of life and manas or mind is actually the controller of all senses that determines the actions of the body. It is responsible for maintaining a balance or harmony between the universal intelligence and human life. In Ayurveda, manas or mind is given the central importance. It is believed that all the phenomena of life or the universe are directly influenced by the 'gunas' or the three primary phases of life. The gunas or the three phases of creation govern the human existence and regulate the minds. These phases generate action, motivation, fascination and inspiration.

Indriya: The Five Senses

The Indriya or the five senses is the third major component of human life defined by the Ayurveda. It is believed that the Indriyas act as a bridge between the atma and the manas. The main work of the Indriyas is to gather information from the outer world. The incoming perceptions from the collected information get relayed to the mind in the form of touch, sound, light, colour, taste and smell, which are the five senses of human body. They have an uplifting influence on the mind. So, if the perceptual information gathered is not of proper quality pr quantity, it will have a negative impact over the mind thus creating an imbalance in the body.

Sharira: The Body

The fourth fundamental part of life is the sharira or the body. In Ayurveda, sharira is not given much significance as compared to the subtler parts of the human life. Body id defined as the vehicle through which the connections of the other parts of the body can be established as a whole.

Ayurveda realizes the deep seated relationship between the nature of the disease as well as the disease process hence the principle of Ayurveda has developed a simultaneous approach to diagnosis and pathology and has termed it as `rogi-roga pariksha`. The principles of Ayurveda offer the proper understanding of the fundamentals of human body and its surroundings.

Diseases in Ayurveda

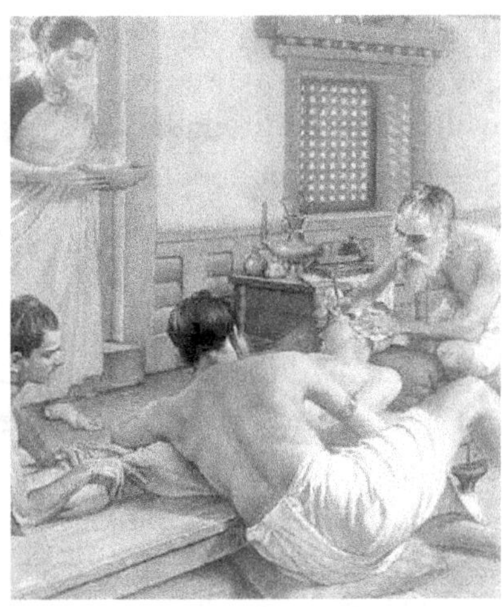

Disease is the state of body and mind in which a person experiences discomfort, pain and injury. The fundamental cause of disease is the imbalance of the three doshas - Vata, Pitta and kapha. When the three doshas are balanced the body experiences health and the state of imbalance or disequilibrium is disease. The imbalance may be due to an increase or decrease in one, two or all the three doshas. The classification of disease in Ayurveda is done in various ways.

Ayurvedic Concept of Disease

The Ayurvedic concept of disease explains pathological condition in terms of doshas, dhatus and malas. The Ayurvedic concept of disease defines two terms, vikruti and prakruti. Vikruti is the abnormal or diseased condition of the body while prakruti refers to the normal physiological and mental state.

Causative Factors of a Disease

According to Ashtang Ayurveda, the causative factors of a disease are an imbalance in any or more of the three doshas (vata, pitta and kapha), the seven dhatus (rasa, rakta, mansa, meda, asthi, majja and shukra), agni and the three malas (mutra, purisha and sweda). The imbalance may be caused by the following conditions: "Asatmendriyarth Samyog", Aama, Pradnyaparadha and Parinama. "Asatmendriyarth Samyog" stands for improper or too much exploitation of the sense organs of vision, sound, smell, sense and touch.

Classification of Disease in Ayurveda

One of the methods of classification of disease in Ayurveda is on the basis of the causative factors. Classified thus, we have three types of diseases: Adhyatmika diseases, Adhibhautika diseases and Adhidaivika diseases. Adhyatmika diseases have their source within the body, and may be further divided into hereditary diseases, congenital disease, and diseases caused by one or more of the doshas or body tissues. Adhibhautika diseases have their source outside the body and incorporate such things as injuries from accidents or mishaps, and according to modern terms, invasions by germs, viruses, and bacteria. Adhidaivika diseases are believed to spring from supernatural sources. This category includes diseases whose exact cause has not yet been found out. It includes ailments cropping up from providential causes, planetary influences, curses and seasonal changes. A more practical classification of disease convenient for treatment classifies the diseases into seven categories. Aadi- bala pravritta refers to those diseases that are transmitted through genes. Human beings are genetically predisposed to fall prey to such diseases. Janma- bala refers to those diseases that are present in the body from birth. Dosha -bala incorporates those diseases that affect the body when the body is suffering from an imbalance of the three doshas, vata, pitta and kapha. Under the category of Sanghata-bala fall those diseases, which are caused by trauma, both physical and mental. Kaala - bala refers to those diseases caused by seasonal changes. Daiva -bala signifies those diseases, which are caused by Gods or spirits. Svabhaava -bala incorporates those diseases that are a part of the natural change of the body with the passage of time. It includes aging and withering of the body.

The classification of disease can also be done as nija, agantuja, sharirik and manasik. Nija refers to endogenous diseases caused by disorder in the doshas. Agantuja stands for exogenous diseases that are caused by external reasons like injuries. Here too the imbalance of doshas does occur but only after the condition of the disease becomes pathological. The diseases caused by physiological disturbances are called sharirik diseases and those, which are a result of psychological disturbances, are known as manasik diseases. Ayurveda also gives the classification of disease according to their curative measures. Thus classified diseases can be Sukhasadhya, Kruchrasadhya, Yapya and Asadhya. Those diseases, which get cured very easily, are categorised under Sukhasadhya. Kruchrasadhya diseases take a lot of time to cure. Those diseases, which recur when the treatment is stopped, fall under the category of Yapya. Asadhya signifies those diseases that are incurable.

Thus, classification of disease is done in many ways in Ayurveda. Such an intensive classification system facilitates proper treatment of diseases.

Parinama in Ayurveda

Parinama refers to abrupt environmental changes, which makes the body vulnerable to disease.Parinama or kala also refers to the effects of time, and the natural physical transformation that are affected as time progresses. In short kala or parinama is defined as "being out of harmony with the rhythms and cycles of Nature". Ayurveda talks about several important cycles at a macrocosmic level, which in turn affects the physiological conditions of human beings.

Pradnyaparadha in Ayurveda

Pradnyaparadha is the improper use of intellect or wisdom that makes the body vulnerable to ailments. This means those thoughtless actions, which are undertaken without determining whether those actions will be detrimental to the proper functioning of the body. These actions may be verbal, mental or physical. The actions stimulated by pradnyaparadha worsen the tridosa system in the body and stimulates the gunas of rajas and tamas creating a pathway through which disease can enter the body.

Chapter 1

Acidity/Heart Burn

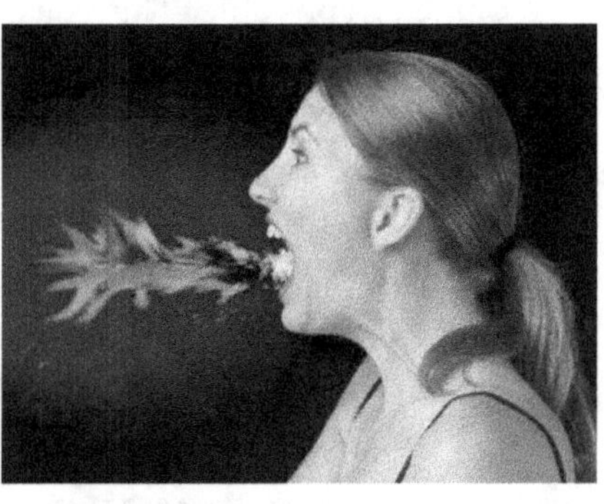

Human blood contains 20 % acid and 80 % alkali. Acids helps to digest food but when acid percentage increases it causes Acidity or heartburn. Symptoms of Acidity are burning pain, sourness in taste, vomiting sensation, coating on the tongue etc. If not treated, Acidity may cause problems like ulcer and other stomach related problems. People with hyper acidity may have regular fever and dizziness. Causes of acidity are eating heavy foods, spicy foods, smoking, alcohol consumption, improper sleep, mental tension, eating without proper chewing, pregnancy, indigestion, menstrual problems etc.

Prevention

Some people have a very acidic body and have weak digestive system. So it is better to prevent acidity by following these instructions.

1. Avoid heavy foods like Kidney beans (Rajma), Black gram (Urad), Milk products, artificial colored sweets, outside junk foods and too much spicy and masala, fried items etc.
2. Eat slowly by chewing properly and take light foods in the night as digestion will be weak in night time.
3. Don't smoke or take alcohol and avoid coffee, tea especially in the empty stomach.

4. Go for walking after meals and don't sleep just after having food and keep some hours of gap between meals and sleep.
5. Don't keep the stomach empty for long time, eat something in between, at least a raisin can do.
6. Sleep properly avoiding all mental tensions, and wear light comfortable cloths while sleeping..
7. Drink lots of water especially in the morning.
8. Drink 1-2 litres of Luke warm water with a pinch of Salt at a time in the morning empty stomach and try to vomit it as much as possible. This is called Kunjal in Yoga. This can be done twice in a week.
9. Avoid raw salads and unripe fruits which are not advisable in Acidity.
10. Instead of eating 2 or 3 heavy meals distribute the same to 5 to 6 light meals a day.

For Acidity taking allopathic medicines wont make you to cut the problem from the root instead it will create some other problems so better use these home remedies for Acidity relief.

Remedies for Acidity/Heart Burn

1. When you have more Acidity, drink 1-2 litres of Luke warm water with a pinch of Salt at a time in the morning empty stomach and try to vomit as much as possible. At the end you feel sourness in the mouth which means you are throwing away the acid. Or you can just drink a glass of water just before brushing and try to take it out just after brushing .
2. Putting a wet cloth (Approximately 8" x 4 ") on the stomach covering naval for a couple of hours gives relief from Acidity.
3. Drinking half glass of Cold milk gives a cooling effect and gives instant relief from Acidity.
4. Mint (Pudina) juice is also a good medicine for Acidity.
5. Tender coconut water taken in empty stomach gives cooling effect and relives Acidity. Daily use of Tender coconut water (2-3) for few months can give permanent relief from Acidity and other stomach related problems.

6. Eating a Plain Ice-cream (Not a flavored or coloured) like vanilla gives instant relief from Acidity.

7. Drinking Falsa (Grewiab subinaequalis) juice or eating Falsa is a best remedy to overcome Acidity and improve digestion.

8. Eating one Clove (Laung) after every meals helps to get relief from Acidity.

9. Drinking Ash gourd (Petha) juice in empty stomach for a month gives relief from hyper Acidity and cures ulcer.

10. Banana makes a good coating on the layers inside the stomach and is a best remedy for curing Acidity.

11. Indian gooseberry (Amla) taken with equal amount of Sugar candy (Mishri) is also a good remedy for Acidity.

12. Potato contains potassium salt which reduces acidity. Eating Boiled Potato helps to get rid of Acidity.

13. Eating Cucumber, Watermelon, Banana helps to get relief from Acidity.

14. Sucking a piece of Jaggery (Gur) or Raisin (Kishmish) gives instant relief from Acidity.

15. Taking some Basil leaves (Tulsi) in the morning helps to overcome Acidity.

16. Lemon juice with hot water taken an hour before meals helps to overcome Acidity. Lemon contains potassium which reduces acid and helps for easy digestion.

17. Having a white Onion with Curd at least for a week cures Acidity.

18. Cumin seeds (Jeera), Coriander (Dhania) , Sugar candy (Mishri) in equal quantities powdered and taken 2 spoons twice a day helps to cure Acidity.

19. Half spoon of Black pepper (Kali mirch) powder taken with Rock salt twice a day helps to get relief from Acidity.

20. Sitting 5 mins in Vajrasan after every meals helps to get relief from Acidity.

21. Eating a Harad (Haritaki, Terminalia chebula) regularly helps to overcome Acidity.
22. One spoon of grinded Carrom (Ajwain) seeds mixed with a spoon of Lemon juice taken with a glass of water gives relief from Acidity.
23. Drinking Carrot juice or eating Raw Carrot regularly helps to overcome Acidity.
24. Drinking Bael juice regularly gives cooling effect and reduces Acidity.
25. Eating Banana with a pinch of Cardamom (Elaichi) powder gives relief from Acidity.

Chapter 2

Acne/Pimples

Acne is a skin problem which mainly happens in teenage. The pimples formed can leave marks later. Though pimples are normal in that age it can increase because of so many factors like improper diet, hormonal imbalance, smoking, alcohol, mental tension, uncleanness, constipation, less water intake etc.

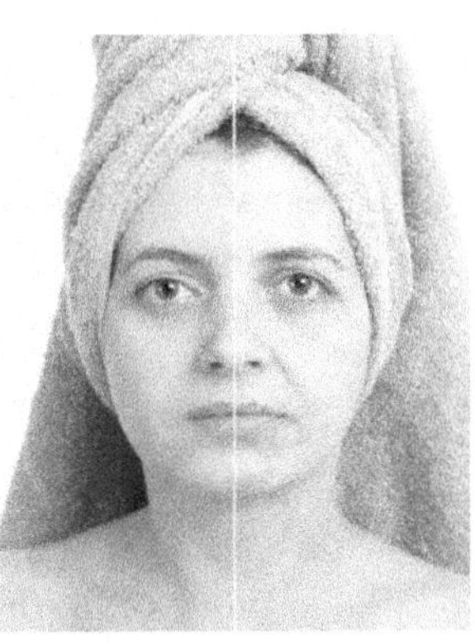

Prevention

1. Drink at least 2-3 litres of water a day and specially 1 to 1.5 litres on empty stomach in the morning.
2. Keep the stomach clean, avoid constipation problem and have fibrous, fruits and raw vegetables.
3. Keep washing face frequently and don't go for soaps, cosmetics which increases Acne problem.
4. Avoid spicy foods, oily and fried items, chocolates, coffee, tea, smoking, alcohol etc
5. Avoid tensions and have a good sleep.

Remedies for Acne and Acne scars

1. Sandalwood paste applied on the face helps to overcome Acne and remove its scars.
2. Cucumber (Kheera) juice mixed with Lemon juice applied on the pimples helps to get relief from Acne and Acne scars.
3. Mint (Pudina) juice applied on the face also helps to get relief from Acne and Acne scars.

4. Water boiled with Neem leaves used for taking steam helps in reducing Acne and Acne scars.
5. Gram flour (Besan) mixed with Buttermilk applied on the face reduces Acne and Acne scars.
6. Raw Papaya (Papita) paste applied on the face helps to cure Acne.
7. Nutmeg (Joy phal) grinded with Milk applied on the face helps a lot in reducing Acne and Acne scars.
8. Powdered Dry Orange skin applied as a paste or Orange skin rubbed on the face helps to remove Acne scars.
9. Water boiled with Neem leaves used for washing face removes extra oil from the face and reduces pimple or Acne.
10. Tomato rubbed on the face or Tomato juice applied on the face helps to remove Acne scars.
11. Aloe Vera (Gwar Patha) is a best medicine for pimples or Acne. Aloe Vera leaf rubbed on the face removes Acne and Acne scars.
12. Carrom seeds (Ajwain) grinded with Curd applied on the face also helps to get rid of Acne or pimples.
13. Fenugreek (Methi) paste also helps in getting rid of Acne and its scars.
14. Basil leaves (Tulsi) rubbed on the face helps to remove Acne scars.
15. Lemon juice applied on the pimples also helps to remove Acne and its scars.
16. Washing face with Tender coconut water is a good remedy to overcome Acne scars.
17. Coriander (Dhania) juice mixed with Lemon juice applied on the face also removes Acne and its scars.

Chapter 3

Anemia

Anemia is nothing but decrease in the concentration of red blood cells in the blood or reduced hemoglobin. Causes of Anemia may be surgery, worm infection, deficiency of iron, folic acid, pregnancy, menstruation problems, lack of nutrition,

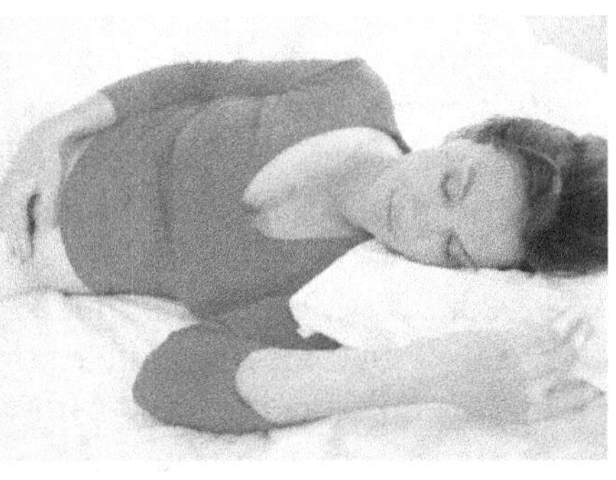

hernia, piles etc. Symptoms of Anemia are weakness, pale face, pale lips and eyes, dizziness, fatigue, constipation etc.

Remedies for Anemia

1. Eat lot of green vegetables especially leafy vegetables like Spinach (Palak), Fenugreek (Menthi), Carrot, Amaranth (red Cholayi) and, Beetroot which are rich in folic acid. Go for citrus fruits like Orange, Sweet lime (Mosambi) which are rich in vitamin C.
2. Honey is a excellent medicine to cure Anemia. Eating a spoon of Honey or taking Honey with Milk twice a day will increase hemoglobin level as well as purify the blood.
3. Dates (Khajur) or Dry Dates (Chuhara) are very helpful in increasing blood level and curing Anemia.
4. Eating Almonds (Badam) everyday also helps to increase blood level and curing Anemia.
5. As Jaggery (Gur) is a good source of iron consume it more instead of sugar which definitely cures Anemia.

6. Eating a Gooseberry (Amla) everyday also helps in improving in blood level and curing Anemia as it is a good source of vitamin C. Also taking 3 spoons of Gooseberry juice with 3 spoons of pure Ghee for 21 days will definitely cures Anemia.

7. Taking Beet root juice or raw Beet root is a excellent medicine for curing Anemia.

8. Spinach (Palak) juice or Tomato juice taken everyday also helps in improving blood level and curing Anemia.

9. Drinking Lemon water with Honey everyday also helps in improving blood level and curing Anemia.

10. Eating a raw Onion or drinking raw Onion juice everyday helps to cure Anemia.

11. Taking 5 milliliter of Ginger juice with old Jaggery (Gur) everyday morning helps to cure Anemia.

12. Pure cows Buttermilk mixed with Sugar Candy (Mishri) taken 3-4 times a day helps to cure Anemia problem.

13. 250 milliliters of cow Milk mixed with 10 gram of pure Ghee, 10 gram of Sugar, 5 gram of Honey, a pinch of Long pepper (Pipple) and a pinch of Black pepper (Kali mirch) taken everyday for 2-3 weeks will definitely cure Anemia.

14. Amrita (Giloy or Tinospora) stem chopped taken 20 gram, Black pepper 10 gram, Garlic 5 gram grinded together and taken around 3 gram with milk everyday morning cures Anemia.

15. Drinking Buttermilk (Chach) made from goats milk for some days also helps to cure Anemia.

16. Drinking Apple juice everyday or eating a Apple (which is a natural source of iron) everyday helps in curing Anemia.

17. Drinking Falsa (Grewiab subinaequalis) juice or eating Falsa fruit is also a good remedy for curing Anemia.

18. Eating Pomegranate (Anar) regularly helps to increase blood level and cures Anemia.

19. Soya bean, Ragi are also said to be very good for Anemia patients if taken in any form.

Chapter 4

Asthma

Asthma is a chronic respiratory disease which causes difficulty in breathing with inflammations in the breathing passage or air ways. Asthma is mainly caused due to allergies.

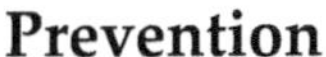

Prevention

1. Keep your stomach clean without constipation problem.
2. Go for walking in a healthy weather, avoid smoke, powerful smells, polluted atmosphere
3. Eat light foods. Don't go for heavy foods, dinner should not be late and heavy. Avoid cold.
4. Don't eat chilled foods, fast foods, chocolates, artificial coloured foods, groundnuts, bananas, water melons.
5. Doing Yoga and Pranayama is definitely helpful and a permanent cure for asthma.

Remedies for Reducing or Curing Asthma

1. Vitamin E is essential for Asthma patients so go for Sprouted wheat, Soya bean, coconut, tomato, grapes, dry fruits etc.
2. Calcium is also essential for Asthma patients, take Milk, Spinach (Palak), Amaranth (Cholayi), Carrot, Gooseberry (Amla), Paneer, Arrow root (Paniphal or Singhada) etc.
3. Two Figs (Anjeer) dipped overnight and taken in the morning for few days helps to cure Asthma.
4. Fenu greek (Menthi) and Carrom seeds (Ajwain) boiled in

water filtered and this decoction mixed with Honey taken thrice a day regularly cures Asthma.

5. One Betel leaf (Pan) put 5 Basil (Tulsi) leaves, one Clove, pinch of Camphor (Kapoor) and fold it. Eat this everyday to cure Asthma.

6. Dry Dates (Chuhara) and Dates (Khajur) both gives strength to lungs which is beneficial for curing Asthma.

7. In one cup of hot water mix one spoon of Lemon juice, two spoons of Honey and a spoon of Ginger juice. Drinking this daily helps to cure Asthma.

8. Garlic juice mixed with Honey or Garlic juice with hot water can be taken everyday which is very good for Asthma patients.

9. One Ounce of Brahmi (Gotu kola) juice taken in the morning for 21 days cures Asthma.

10. Eating Turmeric powder with hot water is a good remedy for curing Asthma.

11. Four Long pepper (Pipple) boiled with a glass of Milk, filtered added Jaggery or Sugar and taking this milk everyday helps in curing Asthma.

12. Wheat grass juice taken everyday is a very good remedy to cure Asthma.

13. Bitter gourd (Karela) is also good for Asthma patients.

14. Drinking Sweet lime (Mosambi) juice with hot water, Cumin (Jeera) powder and dry Ginger powder (Saunth) helps in curing Asthma.

15. Half gram of Alum (Phitkari) with a spoon of Honey taken helps in Asthma.

16. Drinking a spoon of Mint (Pudina) juice with water everyday helps to cure Asthma.

17. Ginger, Long pepper (Pipple) , Black pepper (Kali mirch) in equal quantities powdered and one spoon of this powder taken with Honey everyday cures Asthma.

18. Drinking Honey with hot water thrice a day helps to reduce Asthma.

19. Bael juice with a spoon of Long pepper (Pipple) powder and Honey taken thrice a week cures Asthma.
20. One cup of cow Milk or goat Milk mixed with a spoon of Turmeric powder, Black pepper powder and Sugar taken everyday helps to cure Asthma.
21. Bael leaves boiled in water, filtered and this filtered water taken hot, helps to reduce Asthma.
22. Taking half spoon of Black pepper powder mixed with a spoon of Honey helps in reducing Asthma.
23. Banana leaf burnt and its ash mixed with Honey taken also cures Asthma.
24. Massaging the chest with Mustard (Sarson) oil mixed with Rock helps to get relief from Asthma.

Chapter 5

Bad Body Odour

Bad body odour can be due to many reasons like uncleanness, tight fitting cloths and shoes, stomach disorders, skin infections, consuming non vegetarian food etc. Balanced Diet with lot of fruits, vegetables and drinking more water and taking bath twice a day al these are necessary to control body odour.

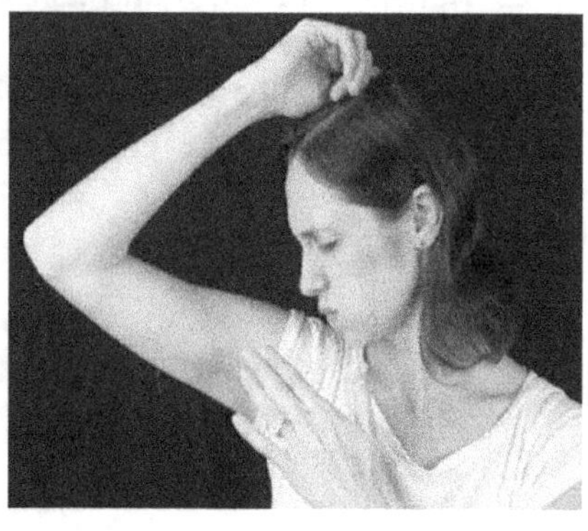

Remedies for Bad Body Odour

1. Applying the paste of Gram flour (Besan) mixed with Curd on the whole body before taking bath cleans and opens the pores which helps in removing bad body odour.
2. Bael leaves dried and powdered then mixed with Shikakai (Soap nut) can be used for taking bath in stead of soap helps to overcome bad body odour.
3. Betel (Pan) leaves grinded with equal quantity of Gooseberry (Amla) and this paste applied on the body before taking bath cures bad body odour.
4. Tamarind (Imli) leaves grinded with Banana tree root and applied on the body before taking bath also helps to overcome bad body odour.
5. Drinking Carrot (Gajar) juice everyday helps to overcome bad body odour problem.

6. After eating onion, garlic, chewing Aniseeds (Sauf) or Dhania or even Mint leaves (Pudina) helps to overcome bad odour.

7. After eating Radish (Muli) eat Jaggery (Gur) and Aniseeds (Sauf) to avoid bad odour.

8. Inhaling or smelling Basil (Tulsi) juice helps to overcome bad odour from nose.

Chapter 6

Bad Breath

Bad breath can be because of many reasons like sinus problem, indigestion, stomach related and lung problems, gum diseases, poor oral hygiene, radiation therapy, hunger, menstrual problems, mouth breathing, dieting, bronchitis, consumption of coffee, tea, tobacco, alcohol etc. Some home remedies have given to stop bad breath .But we suggest you to keep your stomach clean as stomach causes 90 % of problems and bad breath is also related to stomach upsets.

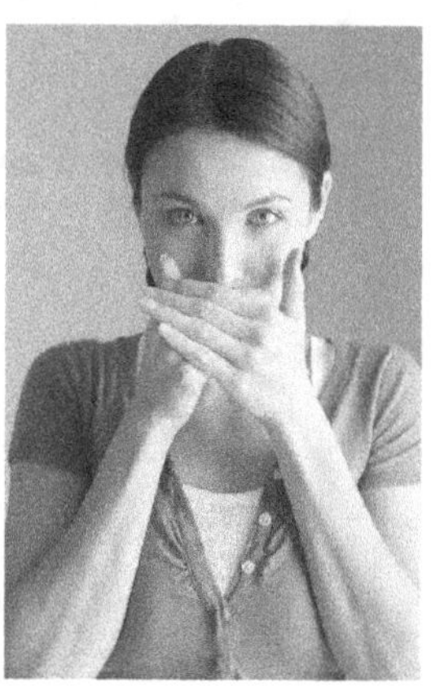

Prevention
1. Eat healthy fibrous foods and avoid constipation problem.
2. Drink lots of water especially in the morning.
3. Don't jump breakfast and don't give much gap for breakfast after you get up.
4. Avoid mouth breathing.
5. Regular flossing, brushing of teeth and cleaning tongue are must.

Remedies for Bad Breath
1. Chewing Basil (Tulsi) leaves everyday helps to stop bad breath problem.
2. Equal quantities of Areca nut (Supari), Garlic and Nut meg (Joy phal) powdered. One spoon of this powder taken with water before sleeping stops bad breath.

3. Pomegranate (Anar) skin can be boiled in water and washing mouth with this water also helps to cure bad breath.

4. Chewing tender Henna (Mehandi) leaves and spitting its juice also helps to stop bad breath problem.

5. Boil some Mint (Pudina) leaves in water and keep drinking this water or just chewing Mint leaves helps to stop bad breath.

6. Durva (Dub, a grass used to worship Lord Ganesha) boiled in water and this filtered water used as a mouth wash also stops bad breath.

7. Ginger juice mixed with hot water can be used as a mouth wash also stops bad breath.

8. Eating Californian raisin (Monakka) daily for 15 days helps to cure bad breath.

9. Washing mouth with Lemon water which also helps to stop bad breath.

10. Eating roasted Cumin seeds (Jeera) or Carrom (Ajwain) seeds or Carrom leaf or Aniseeds (Sauf) also helps to stop bad breath.

11. Sucking a Cardamom (Elaichi) or Clove (Laung) after meals also helps to stop bad breath.

12. Long pepper (Pipple) powdered and taken with Honey regularly helps to stop bad breath.

Chapter 7

Baldness

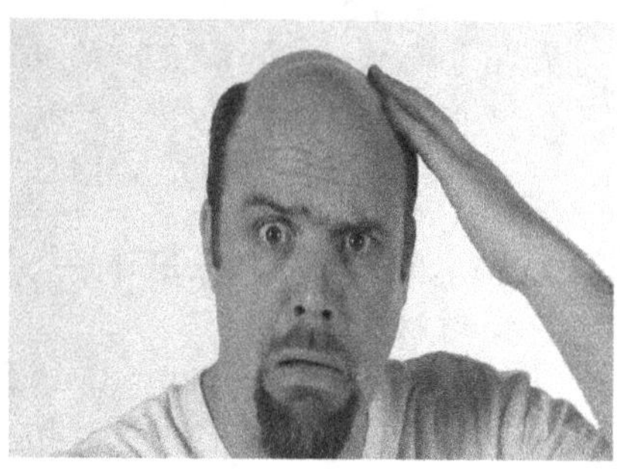

Main causes of baldness are mental tensions, fungal infections, thyroid problem, hormonal changes, chemotherapy, Blood thinners, menopause, heredity etc. By natural home remedies we can overcome this baldness problem.

Remedies for Baldness

1. Pomegranate leaves grinded and this paste applied on the scalp regularly helps to overcome baldness problem.
2. Applying Lemon juice on the scalp helps in growing new hairs and thus helps in curing baldness.
3. Applying Onion paste regularly on the balding area helps in growing new hairs and thus helps in curing baldness.
4. Applying Coriander (Dhania) paste regularly on the balding area helps in growing new hairs and thus helps in curing baldness.
5. Banana pulp meshed with Lemon juice applied on the scalp regularly helps to overcome baldness problem.
6. Applying Neem oil on the balding area for some period helps in growing new hairs and thus helps in curing baldness.

Bed Wetting/Enuresis

Bed wetting is natural in children up to age 5 or 6. But it continues in some children even after this age. Some home made remedies are as below.

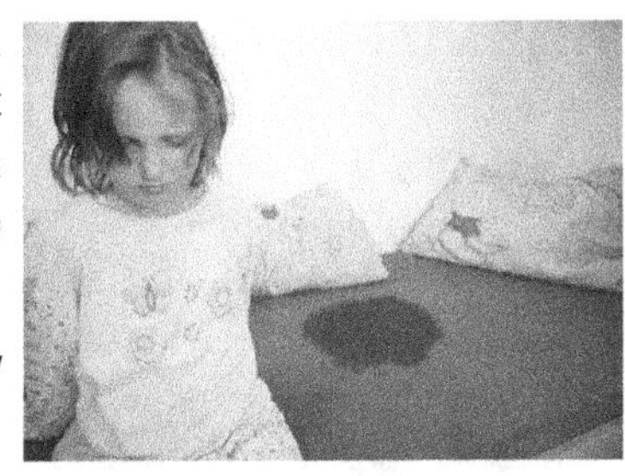

Remedies for Bed Wetting/Enuresis

1. Californian raisin (Monakka) can be given in the night before going to bed cures bed wetting problem.
2. Giving a spoon of Honey before sleeping helps in curing bed wetting problem.
3. Giving 2 Walnuts (Akhroat) with few Raisins (Kishmish) everyday helps to cure bed wetting problem.
4. Gooseberry (Amla) with Sugar candy (Mishri) or Gooseberry Morabba given everyday helps in curing bed wetting problem.
5. Black berry (Jamun) seeds powder given with hot water helps in curing bed wetting problem.
6. Dry dates (Chuhara) given in night with Milk also helps to overcome bed wetting problem.

Chapter 9

Burning Urine/Dysuria

Dysuria is a common complaint in ladies with burning and pain during urination and frequent urge for urination. Sometimes it is unbearable and person cannot tolerate burning. Some home remedies have given which definitely helps to cure burning urine problem. Causes of burning urine are excessive heat in the body, urinary infections, consuming more chilly, less water intake, more sweating, very hot weather etc.

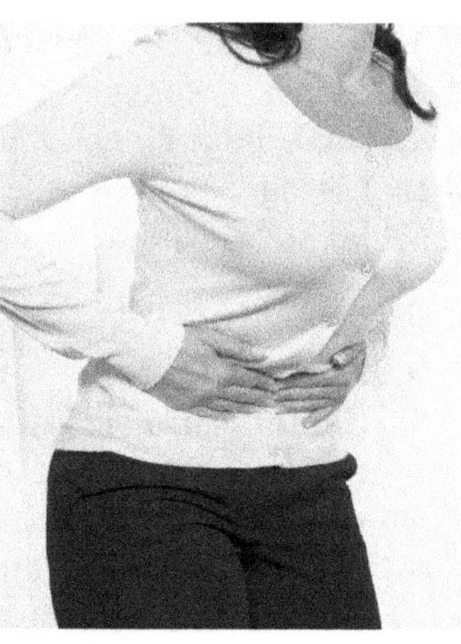

Remedies for Burning Urine/Dysuria

1. Drinking lots of water especially hot water is the best remedy to throw out the infectious material and heat from the body and in curing Dysuria.
2. Drinking Tender Coconut Water mixed with Jaggery (Gur) and half spoon of Coriander (Dhania) powder helps in curing Dysuria.
3. Drinking Cucumber (Kheera) juice twice a day helps to stop burning and pain during urination and cures Dysuria.
4. Mix a spoon of Coriander (Dhania) powder in water in the night. Filter it in the morning and add Sugar candy (Mishri) to this decoction. Drinking this helps in curing burning urine or Dysuria.
5. Drinking a spoon of Radish (Muli) juice in the morning also helps in curing Dysuria .

6. Cardamom (Elaichi) powder taken with Milk helps to cure Dysuria.

7. Drinking Aloe Vera (Gwar patha) juice is a very good remedy to cure Dysuria.

8. Around 10 gram of old Tamarind (Imli) pulp mixed with Tender coconut water or Tamarind pulp mixed with water can be taken to cure Dysuria.

9. Drinking Carrot juice every day helps to cure burning urine problem or Dysuria.

10. Dry Ginger (Saunth) Powder and Sugar candy (Mishri) mixed with Milk taken twice a day also helps to cure Dysuria.

11. Taking Drumstick leaves (Muranka Bhaji) grinded and mixed with Jaggery also helps to cure Dysuria.

12. Drinking Honey with water every 2 hrs will cure Dysuria.

13. Luke warm water mixed with Lemon juice taken also helps to cure Dysuria.

14. Four spoons of Gooseberry (Amla) juice mixed with a spoon of Sugar candy (Mishri) powder taken twice a day helps to cure Dysuria.

15. Dip few Raisins (Kishmish), Gooseberry (Amla) powder, Sugar candy (Mishri) in the night and drinking this water in the morning is a best remedy to cure Dysuria.

16. Cardamom (Elaichi) powder, Roasted Cumin (Jeera) powder and Sugar mixed in pure Butter can be taken twice a day helps to cure Dysuria.

17. Taking a spoon of Durva (Dub, a grass used to worship Lord Ganesha) juice with a glass of fresh Milk also helps in curing Dysuria.

18. Drinking Water melon or Bael juice helps in reducing burning sensation and cures Dysuria.

19. Putting a Wet cloth on the naval reduces stomach heat and gives relief from burning during urination.

20. Ridge gourd (Touri) taken in any form is effective in reducing burning and curing Dysuria.

21. Jo (Barley) boiled in water and cooled and consumed makes cooling effect on the body and reduces burning and Dysuria.

Chapter 10

Burns

The first and foremost in burns is to reduce the temperature of the burnt area. For this, put lots of chilled water or dip the affected area into chilled water at least for 15-30 minutes. Keep yourself hydrated. Drink plenty of water to make your body in harmony. The burns will take up the electrolytes in terms of water from your body. For this, one can go for the lemon juice with sugar and pinch of salt. It is also effective natural cure for burns.

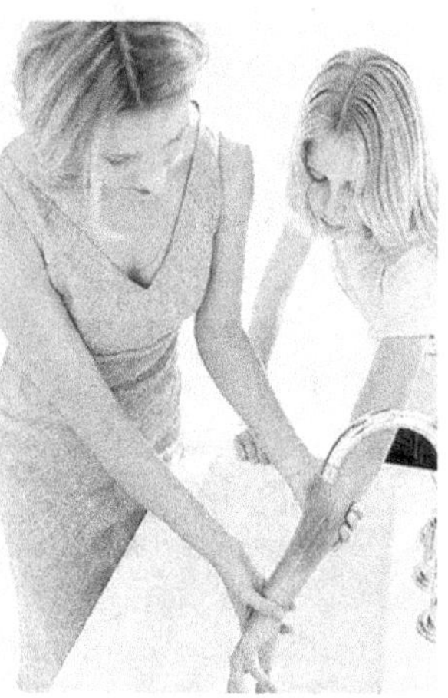

Remedies for Burns

1. Putting cold water immediately on the burned area till the burning sensation reduces helps in reducing the effect of burn and prevents formation of blisters. Keep drinking water, milk, curd etc.
2. Applying Honey regularly on the burns helps to reduce burning and heals faster and also removes burning scars.
3. Harad (Haritaki) powder mixed with Honey can be applied on the burns reduces burning and heals faster.
4. Raw Potato juice or Potato paste applied on the burns helps to reduce burning and heals faster.
5. Turmeric paste applied on the burned wounds reduce burning and heals faster.
6. Applying Ghee on the burns helps to reduce burning and heals faster.

7. Mango leaves burnt and its ashes sprinkled on the burns heals faster.

8. Mustard oil (Sarson ka teil) applied on the burns help to avoid blisters.

9. Aloe Vera (Gwar Patha) juice applied regularly on the burns helps to reduce burning, faster healing and removing scars.

10. Sesame seeds (Til) grinded and applied as a thick paste on the burns heals faster and reduce burning.

11. Applying thick paste of Sugar on the burns helps to reduce burning .

12. Banana pulp applied on the burns helps to reduce burning sensation.

13. Carrot grinded and its paste applied on the burns helps to reduce burning sensation.

14. Applying thick paste of Salt on the burns helps to avoid blisters.

15. Applying thick paste of Onion on the burns helps to reduce burning and heals faster.

16. Applying thick paste of Fenu greek seeds (Menthi) on the burns helps to reduce burning and prevents blister formation.

17. Basil (Tulsi) juice with Coconut oil applied on the burns helps to heal faster.

18. Applying Glycerin on the burns reduces burning.

Chapter 11

Cancer

Cancer is a fatal disease in which growth of abnormal cells are uncontrolled resulting in tumor, mass, slowly destroying surrounding tissues. Cancer can spread from its original sites to other parts of the body or blood stream. Normal Cancers are breast Cancer, brain Cancer, blood Cancer, lung 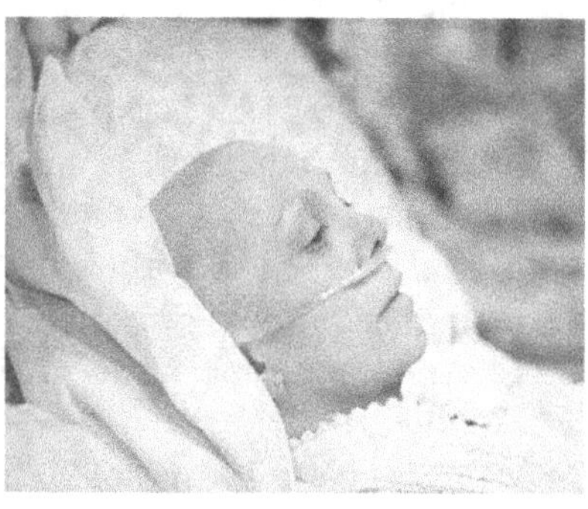 Cancer, skin Cancer, thyroid Cancer, prostate Cancer, pancreatic Cancer, bladder Cancer, kidney Cancer, colo-rectal Cancer, mouth Cancer, bone Cancer etc.

Symptoms of Cancers are delayed healing of wounds, tumor or lumps unusual bleeding or discharge in ladies, indigestion and difficulty to swallow, sore throat, constant fever, chills, changes in the color of moles, weakness, loss of appetite and weight loss, constipation, diarrhoea, cough etc.

Prevention

1. Avoid cosmetics which include harmful chemicals which affect skin and cause skin Cancer.
2. Avoid smoking and tobacco consumption which may cause mouth Cancer or lung Cancer or throat Cancer.
3. Although we cannot cure Cancer by our home remedies we can reduce its effect or we can prevent Cancer if followed regularly.

Remedies for Cancer

- Chewing 3-5 Basil (Tulsi) leaves everyday morning helps to prevent all type of Cancers.
- Drinking Wheat grass juice every day morning is a very helpful remedy which reduce Cancer effects and also prevents Cancer.
- Drinking Bael juice or eating Bael pulp is beneficial in blood Cancer and bone Cancers.
- Drinking own Urine everyday morning also helps to reduce Cancer effects.
- Drinking Cauliflower (Phool gobi) juice in the morning helps to prevents and reduce Cancer effects.
- Drinking Carrot juice twice a day empty stomach helps to reduce Cancer effects.
- Carrot juice mixed with small quantity of Spinach (Palak) juice taken everyday helps to reduce Cancer effects.
- Using Cabbage, Cauliflower, Lemon, Carrot, Sweet lime (Mosambi), Lentils (Sabut dals) regularly in meals prevents and reduce Cancer effects.
- Drinking Durva (Dub, a grass used to worship Lord Ganesha) juice with Honey regularly reduces Cancer effects.

Chapter 12

Chickenpox

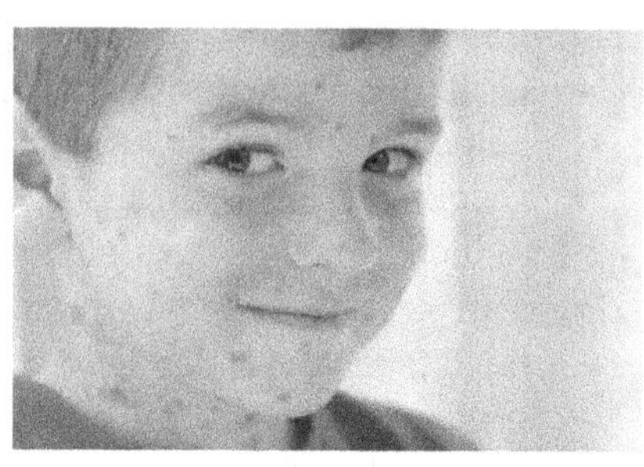

Chickenpox is a viral infection and highly contagious disease. The symptoms are high fever, loss of appetite, headache, stomach ache and red rashes on the skin. These rashes or blisters may vary from 250 to 500 in numbers when chickenpox reaches its peak.

Remedies for Chickenpox

1. Salt, chilies, ghee, oil, spices (Masala) should not be taken at least 15 days after getting the Chickenpox symptoms. The food should be very light and easily digestible. Remember that salt will cause itching in rashes during Chickenpox so avoid using salt. Don't eat banana, brinjal, sweet pumpkin for some days even after the Chickenpox is completely cured. Don't touch the rashes and if the itching is intolerable one can use neem leaves to itch. Avoid taking bath for 15 days or till the rashes are completely subsides and dries up.

2. Boil Neem leaves in water for 10 minutes and filter it. Drink a glass of this decoction in the empty stomach for 3 days of the starting of the Chickenpox.

3. For taking bath after 15 days, Boil some Neem leaves in water for sometime and use this water for bath. But rashes should not be rubbed.

4. Drink lot of water to avoid dehydration which is a common problem during Chickenpox.
5. Drink Milk in sufficient quantity during Chickenpox but don't drink in the empty stomach which can create gas.
6. To get rid of Chickenpox scars it is very important that rashes should not be touched. Remember that it takes 1-2 month for the rash scars to get the original colours as the time required for the pigmentation is more. Still following these home remedies can be used to get rid of Chickenpox scars. But remember not to apply anything till the rashes dries.
7. Applying Honey on the Chickenpox scars helps to reduce them.
8. Applying Sandal wood oil (Sandalwood powder boiled with Coconut oil and filtered) or pure Coconut oil also helps to reduce Chickenpox scars.

13. Cholera

Cholera is an acute fatal infectious disease of intestinal infection caused by unhygienic contaminated water or food and characterized by watery diarrhoea, nausea, vomiting, dehydration, high fever, cramps, suppression of urine, rapid heart rate, dry skin, excessive thirst and weakness and can even cause death.

Though we cannot cure Cholera fully by this home remedies these helps to reduce Cholera effects.

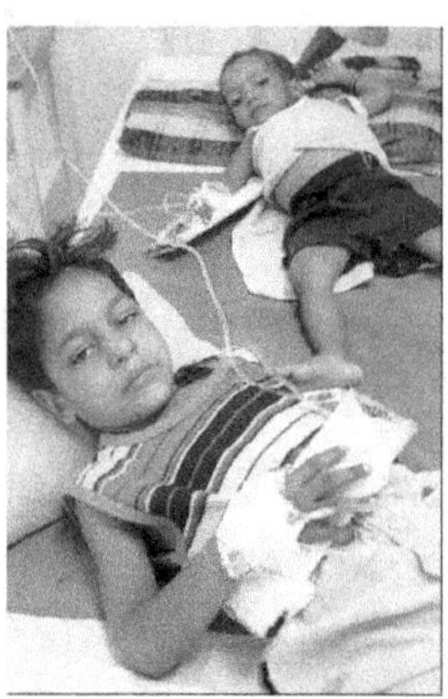

Remedies for Cholera

1. Eating Onion regularly helps to prevent Cholera and also reduce Cholera effects.
2. Drinking Lemon juice helps to kill Cholera bacteria and reduce Cholera effects.
3. Eating Garlic helps to reduce Cholera effects.
4. Drinking Bitter gourd (Karela) juice also helps to reduce Cholera effects.
5. Cardamom (Elaichi), Tamarind (Imli), Mint leaves (Pudina), Black pepper (Kali mirch) all grinded together and slowly sucking this mixture reduce Cholera effects. Especially it reduces vomiting and watery diarrhoea.
6. Drinking sour Butter milk (Chach) reduces vomiting and diarrhoea during Cholera.

14. Cholesterol

Cholesterol is an abundant fatty substance found in animal tissues and various foods and is critically important. Although some Cholesterol is obtained from the diet most Cholesterol is made in the liver and other tissues. Elevated Cholesterol level leads to blockage in arteries, heart problems etc.

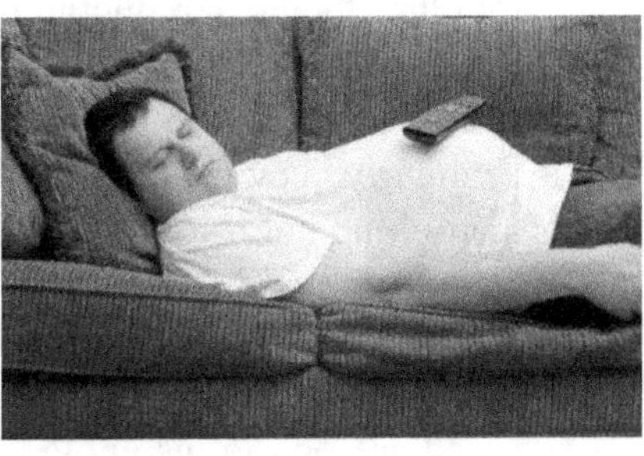

Prevention

1. Avoid Maida based products which tends to upset the insulin balance which leads to an increase in Cholesterol.
2. Ghee, Paneer, Butter, Cream, Fried items should be avoided.
3. Non vegetarian food especailly red meats should be avoided.
4. Liver is the seat of Cholesterol metabolism and Alcohol affects the liver so alcohol should be avoided.
5. Aerated drinks, Fast foods should be avoided.

Remedies for Cholesterol

1. People suffering from high Cholesterol should drink at least 8 to 10 glasses of water per day as it stimulates the activity of skin and kidneys thereby reducing excessive Cholesterol from the system.
2. Regularly eating Curd helps in reducing bad Cholesterol.
3. Regularly eating raw Garlic helps in reducing Cholesterol level.

4. Regular drinking of a decoction of Coriander (Dhania) seeds helps to stimulate kidneys and reduce Cholesterol level.
5. Regularly eating Ginger helps in reducing Cholesterol level as ginger helps in blood circulation and keeps liver healthy.
6. Regular physical exercises like bicycling, swimming, jogging etc are helpful in improving blood circulation and enhancing the good Cholesterol level.
7. Finely chopped Onion pieces mixed with a cup of Buttermilk along with half spoon of Black pepper (Kali mirch) taken regularly helps in reducing bad Cholesterol level.
8. Eat plenty of fruits with their skin as fruit skin contains pectin which is a soluble fibre that blinds Cholesterol.
9. Regularly chewing Sweet Neem (Curry patta) or using them in cooking helps to reduce Cholesterol level.
10. Regularly eating Fenugreek (Menthi) seeds or Fenugreek sprouts helps in reducing Cholesterol level.
11. Eating unprocessed fibre rich wheat flour, whole wheat bread are rich in insoluble fibre which helps in flushing out oil from the intestine.
12. Soya flour, Barley, Oat all are helpful in reducing Cholesterol level.

Chapter 15

Cold/Running Nose

Cold can be due to many reasons like allergies, Cold weather, nasal problems, sudden change in temperature, Drinking water or facing air conditioner as soon as coming from hot sun, rain wetting, pollution, etc.

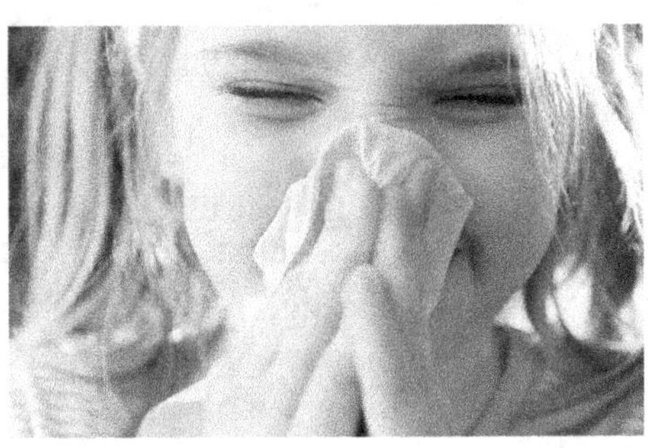

Remedies for Cold/Running Nose

1. Vitamin C deficiency can often cause Cold problems. So go for rich natural source of vitamin C like Oranges, Gooseberries (Amla), Sweet lime (Mosambi), Grapes, Guava (Amrud) etc.

2. Eating hot Gram flour halva helps in controlling running nose instantly and effectively. Roast Gram flour (Besan) with Ghee (Butter oil) till it changes to light brown color, then add water and Sugar and cook for few minutes.

3. Eating a small piece of Onion (Pea size) or sucking a piece of Clove (Laung) helps to get instant relief from cold or running nose.

4. Ragi mixed with Turmeric powder sprinkled on the burning coal and the fumes inhaled cures nose blockage or cold very fast.

5. Turmeric powder sprinkled on the burning coal and the fumes inhaled (but after that don't drink water for 5 hours) cures nose blockage, cold very fast.

6. Boiling Long pepper (Pipple) in the Milk with Sugar candy (Mishri) and drinking this milk helps in curing running nose or cold.

7. Eating a Apple everyday before meals cures and prevents running nose or cold .

8. Dry Ginger powder (Saunth) mixed with old Jaggery (Gur) taken twice a day helps to cure running nose or cold.

9. Milk boiled with Ginger, Black pepper (Kali mirch), Basil (Tulsi) leaves, Cloves (Laung), Red Sugar candy (Mishri) or Jaggery is very useful in curing Cold. This should be taken hot before going to bed, and cover the body to preserve body heat, for few days.

10. Few drops of fresh Neem leaves juice put in the nostrils cures running nose or cold easily.

11. Taking steam with Eucalyptus oil drops helps in curing cold or nose blockage.

12. Rubbing the whole body using Salt while taking bath helps to cure cold or running nose.

13. Eating Sesame seeds (Til) roasted with ghee and mixed with Jaggery helps in curing running nose during winter.

14. Black pepper powder, Ginger juice and Basil juice mixed with Honey taken thrice a day cures running nose or cold.

15. Making Tea with few Mint (Pudina) leaves or with Ginger or with Basil leaves and drinking cures running nose or cold.

16. Figs (Anjeer) boiled in water and this hot water taken twice a day cures cold or running nose.

17. Taking Garlic in any form helps in curing running nose, sneeze or cold.

18. Betel leaf with a Clove can be taken to cure running nose or cold.

19. Aniseeds (Sauf) and Cloves boiled in water for 10 minutes added Sugar and filtered. Drinking this hot decoction helps to cure cold or running nose.

20. Eating half spoon of Turmeric powder and drinking hot water for few days helps to overcome running nose or cold.

21. Drinking hot water with Lemon juice and Honey in the night helps to overcome running nose or cold.
22. Smelling Asafetida (Hing) helps to reduce cold or running nose.
23. Tamarind (Imli) leaves boiled in water for few minutes and filtered. Taking this decoction also cures cold or running nose.
24. Make a slit in one Onion and fill Turmeric powder in the slit. Roast this Onion on a burning coal and eat before going to bed. Avoid drinking water whole night which helps in curing cold or running nose.
25. Applying Castor oil (Erand ka teil) on the centre of the head helps in curing running nose due to excessive heat in the body.
26. Drinking tender coconut water in the day time helps in curing running nose due to excessive heat in the body.
27. Drinking a spoon of Betel leaves (Pan) juice helps to cure cold or running nose especially in children.
28. Drinking a spoon of Carrom Leaf (Ajwain) juice mixed with Honey helps to cure cold or running nose especially in children .
28. Nut Meg (Joy phal) paste with honey taken helps to cure cold or running nose especially in children .
29. Adding few drops of Doctors brandy in hot milk and given to children helps in curing cold or running nose.

16. Constipation

The causes of Constipation are irregular meals, excessive eating, lack of rest, lack of physical activity, mental tensions, lack of sleep, lack of water intake, smoking, weak intestine, weak digestive system, irregular sleeping habits, consumption of too much coffee or tea, side effects of allopathic medicines etc. People take anema which is only a temporary relief but causes some other problems later on. So it is advisable to use home remedies to overcome Constipation problem.

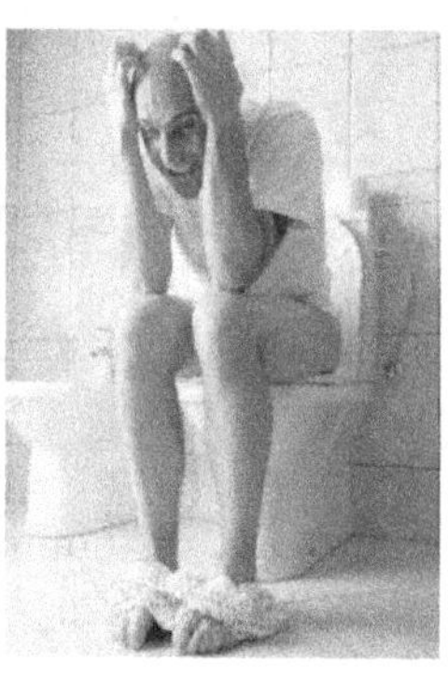

Remedies for Constipation

1. Eating a Harad (Terminalia chebula, Haritaki) everyday helps to overcome Constipation.
2. Taking a spoon of Triphala (Triphala is composed of Harad (Haritaki), Indian gooseberries (Amla) and Behada (Bibhitaki)) every night before going to bed helps to clear the stomach next morning and cures Constipation problem.
3. Massaging the stomach everyday night with Mustard (Sarson) oil helps to cure Constipation problem.
4. Eating Lentil (Masoor dal) regularly helps to clear the stomach and cures Constipation problem.
5. Drinking at least 8 glasses of water per day preferably hot water in the morning helps to cure Constipation.
6. Eating Watermelon (Tarbooj) regularly for few days helps to cure Constipation problem.

7. Drinking raw Spinach juice (Palak) for few days gives permanent relief from Constipation.

8. Eating a ripe Fig (Anjeer) in the night or 5 dried figs boiled with Milk taken before going to bed helps to overcome Constipation.

9. Eating a ripe Papita (Papaya) before going to bed gives relief from Constipation problem.

10. Eating one raw Onion with every meals helps to cure Constipation problem.

11. Radish (Muli) taken with Salt and Black pepper (Kali mirch) clears the stomach and gives relief from Constipation.

12. Hot water with Lemon juice taken in the night gives relief from Constipation.

13. Using Garlic (Lehsun) regularly in cooking helps to get relief from Constipation.

14. Taking Guava (Amrud) with seeds provides roughage to diet and it acts as a laxative in the intestine. It should be taken only before meals to get relief from Constipation.

15. Tomato is also said to be very good for Constipation which helps in cleaning the stools which are sticking in the intestine.

16. Using Fenugreek leaves (Menthi) in meals also helps to reduce Constipation.

17. Eating 250 grams of Fresh Carrot (Gajar) everyday helps to increase appetite and reduce Constipation.

18. Drinking Wheat grass juice regularly helps to overcome Constipation problem.

19. Bitter gourd (Karela) juice taken regularly or eating Bitter gourd helps to overcome Constipation problem.

20. Eating a spoon of powdered Aniseed (Sauf) with hot water in the night helps to cure Constipation.

21. Using Amaranth (Cholayi) regularly in meals also helps to overcome Constipation.

22. Buttermilk (Chach) taken with Carrom seeds (Ajwain) helps to overcome Constipation.

23. Drinking 2-3 drops of Castor oil (Erand) with Milk in the night helps to overcome Constipation.
24. A spoon of Ginger juice boiled with water taken regularly helps to overcome Constipation.
25. Eating raw Cabbage (Patta gobi) everyday helps to overcome Constipation.
26. Drinking Hot milk with Flea seeds (Isabgol) in the night helps to overcome Constipation.
27. Taking half spoon of Black pepper powder mixed with pure Ghee which helps the stick stool to loosen. Later drink hot milk which helps to clear the stomach and cure Constipation.
28. Eating Grapes everyday also helps to overcome Constipation.
29. Eating Bael fruit or drinking Bael juice everyday helps to overcome Constipation as Bael is a good laxative and having more cooling effect on the body.
30. Sprouted Green gram (Moong) is a good remedy to relieve from Constipation.
31. Eat one ripe Banana before going to bed everyday to avoid Constipation.
32. Ripe Banana pulp mixed with Curd taken everyday helps to get relief from Constipation.
33. Eating a ripe Mango after meals helps to get relief from Constipation.
34. Eating raw Beetroot everyday helps to overcome Constipation.
35. Few drops of Castor oil mixed with a spoon of Lemon juice taken in the night helps to cure Constipation.

17. Cough

Common Cough can be due to dust allergies, nasal problems, cold etc. We have given home remedies for common Cough. Severe and prolonged Cough can be symptoms of many diseases like tuberculoses, lung related problems etc.

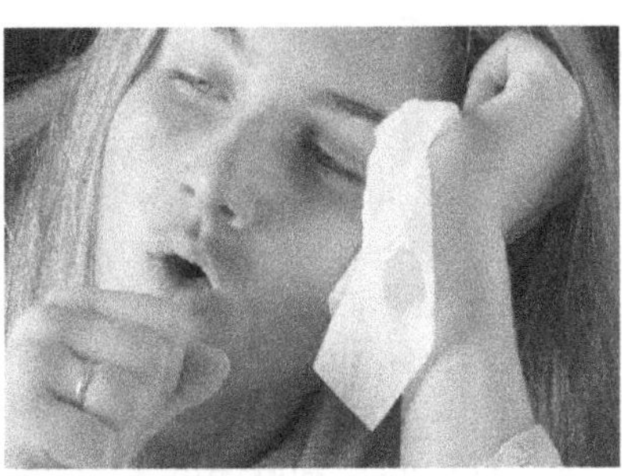

Remedies for Cough

1. Ginger grinded and this paste cooked with Jaggery (Gur) and small quantity of Ghee can be made into small balls and can be stored for few days. Sucking this ball while having Cough is a very good remedy for curing Cough.

2. Milk boiled with Ginger, Black pepper (Kali mirch), Basil (Tulsi) leaves, Cloves (Laung), Red Sugar candy (Mishri) or Jaggery is very useful in curing Cough. After drinking this milk cover the body and take rest for sometime. This can be repeated for few days.

3. Long pepper (Pipple), Black pepper, Almonds (Badam), Red Sugar candy (Mishri) powdered and mixed together and a tea spoon of this mixture taken everyday helps to cure Cough.

4. Basil (Tulsi) juice taken with Sugar candy (Mishri) helps to relieve from Cough, cold, fever.

5. Sucking a piece of Sugar candy or Black pepper or Ginger or Turmeric or Cinnamon gives instant relief and slowly

reduces Cough.

6. One fourth spoon of Black pepper (Kali mirch) powder mixed with Ginger juice and Honey taken once in 2 hours reduces Cough within a day.

7. 4-5 Black Basil leaves and one Betel leaf (Pan) with 2 Cloves (Laung) grinded together and taken will also cure Cough.

8. A spoon of Basil juice and Garlic juice with Honey or Basil juice with Honey taken once in 2 hours helps to cure Cough.

9. Harad (Haritaki) paste applied on the chest helps to reduce Cough.

10. Gargling with hot water and Salt helps to clear phlegm (Balgum) and reduces Cough.

11. Bael pulp without seeds taken with Jaggery reduces Cough and phlegm (Balgum).

12. Basil juice, Onion juice, Ginger juice, Honey mixed together and taking a spoon of this juice once in an hour helps to cure Cough.

13. Turmeric and Black pepper boiled with Milk, filtered and this Milk taken twice a day helps to cure Cough.

14. Sucking a small piece of raw Onion or raw Garlic helps to reduce Cough.

15. Eating an Apple regularly for a week cures Cough completely.

16. Cinnamon (Dalchini) and Black pepper boiled in water and filtered and this decoction taken with Honey cures Cough and reduces phlegm (Balgum).

17. Carrom seeds (Ajwain), Fenugreek seeds (Menthi) boiled with water, filtered and this decoction taken with Honey reduces Cough and phlegm (Balgum).

18. Gooseberry (Amla) powder taken with Honey cures Cough.

19. Gooseberry grinded with Coriander (Dhania) leaves taken helps to cure dry Cough.

20. Eating Figs (Anjeer) helps to reduce phlegm (Balgum).

21. Sesame seeds (Til) and Sugar candy (Mishri) boiled in water for 10 minutes filtered and this decoction taken thrice a day helps to cure Cough.

22. Aniseeds (Sauf), Carrom seeds (Ajwain) boiled in water, filtered and this decoction mixed with Honey taken thrice a day helps to get relief from Cough.
23. Tea made with Ginger and Mint (Pudina) helps to cure Cough.
24. Violet tender Brinjal (Byangan) boiled and taken regularly helps to reduce Cough problem.
25. Lemon piece filled with Black pepper (Kali mirch) powder and Salt sucked slowly reduces Cough.
26. Carrom leaves (Ajwain) grinded with Garlic can be taken as a chutney to cure Cough.
27. Four spoons of Onion juice mixed with a spoon of Honey taken regularly cures Cough.
28. 10 grams of Ginger, Long pepper (Pipple), Black pepper each, with 30 grams of Glycyrriza glabra (Jyeshta madhu) powdered and taken one spoon with Honey thrice a day cures severe Cough.
29. Equal quantities of Harad (Haritaki), Gooseberry, Glycyrriza glabra (Jyeshta madhu) powdered and one spoon of this powder taken with one spoon of Sugar with Milk thrice a day cures severe Cough.
30 grams of Glycyrriza glabra (Jyeshta madhu) powdered and boiled with Milk for 10 minutes, filtered and this Milk taken with Honey thrice a day helps to cure severe Cough.
31. Glycyrriza glabra (Jyeshta madhu) powder boiled with Milk, added with Sugar, filtered and taken helps to get relief from Cough.
32. Raisin (Kishmish), Black pepper, Licorice (Mulethi) in equal quantities powdered and taking a pinch of this powder thrice a day helps to cure severe Cough.
33. Maalbar (Adulasa, adusoge) leaf juice with Honey and Rock salt taken twice a day helps to cure severe Cough.

Dandruff

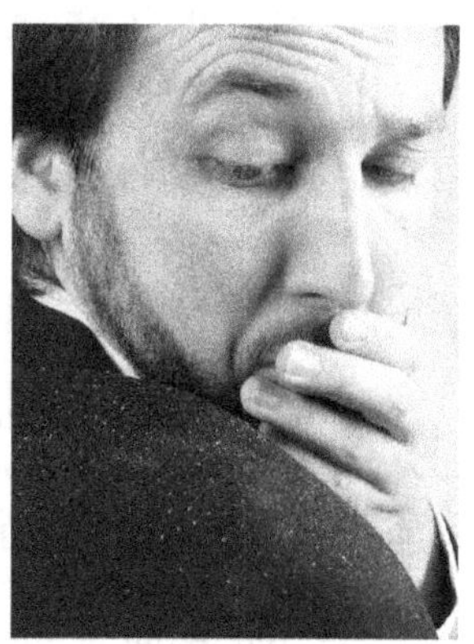

Dandruff is dry flakes of dead skin on the scalp which results in itching, hair loss, damaged hair, skin problems etc. The causes of dandruff are uncleanness, mental tension, fever, infection, excessive use of shampoos, hormonal problems, Eating lots of fried items, chocolates etc.

The shampoos, soaps are harmful to the hair and they cannot completely cures dandruff so it is better to use home made remedies to overcome dandruff problem.

Remedies for Dandruff

1. Fenugreek (Menthi) paste applied on the scalp an hour before taking bath helps to overcome Dandruff problem.
2. Applying Lemon juice on the scalp 10 minutes before taking head bath helps to remove Dandruff.
3. Sour Curd applied on the scalp an hour before taking bath helps to get rid of Dandruff.
4. Reetha (Soap nut) used for washing hair helps to get relief from Dandruff.
5. Indian Gooseberries (Amla) paste applied on the scalp before taking bath helps to get relief from Dandruff.
6. Hibiscus leaves boiled in small quantity of water and used along with Shikakai as a hair wash instead of soap, shampoo helps in reducing Dandruff problem. This is a natural hair conditioner.

7. Gram flour (Besan) mixed with Curd applied on the scalp before bath helps to remove Dandruff.

8. Boiled Beetroot leaves used for washing hairs helps to get rid of Dandruff.

9. Regular oil massage on the scalp helps to get relief from Dandruff.

10. Neem paste or Sweet Neem (Curry patta) paste mixed with Basil (Tulsi) paste applied on the scalp helps to remove Dandruff.

11. Grinded Pigeon pea (Arhar dal) applied on the scalp before taking bath helps to remove Dandruff.

12. Applying crushed raw Papaya (Papita) paste on the scalp 10 minutes before taking bath is very helpful. This process assists in the exfoliation of dandruff flakes and slows down fungal growth. Papaya contains enzyme Papain which is very helpful in reducing dandruff and hair fall problem.

Chapter 19

Diabetes

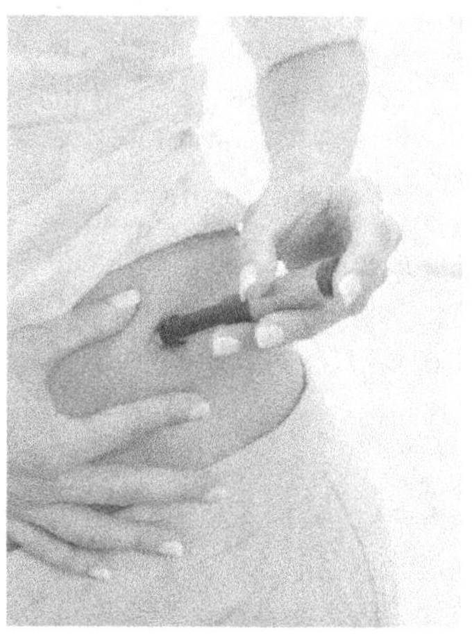

Diabetes is a condition in which body is not able to maintain the blood sugar level and it goes beyond normal and excretion of extra glucose in the urine. Symptoms of Diabetes are too much thirst, too much hunger, frequent urination, skin problems, blurred vision, exhaustion, constipation, very slow healing of wounds, headache, itching, giddiness, sudden weight loss etc. Causes of diabetes are heredity, obesity, mental tension, too much television watching, age, pregnancy, virus which obstructs insulin production, etc.

Diabetic patients should avoid sugar intake in any form. If they are too much urged to eat sweet then can take small quantity of Honey. Rice contains starch and to be avoided. Eat lot of green vegetables, sprouts, dry fruits. Drink lot of water in the morning. Sleep adequately, treat constipation etc.

Remedies for Diabetes

1. Rotis made up of Ragi, Ragi soups, Ragi balls, Ragi in milk can be used. Ragi used in any form is beneficial in Diabetes.
2. Eating a cup of home made Curd helps to slow down the progression of Diabetes. Bacteria's contained in curd can bring about a delaying effect on the progress of Diabetes induced by high fructose administration.

3. Taking Bitter gourd (Karela) juice or Bitter gourd in any form helps to control Diabetes.

4. Black berries (Jamun) seeds powdered and taken regularly and also eating Black berries helps to control Diabetes.

5. Pieces of stem chopped from Red Kino tree (Honne) boiled in water, filtered and this decoction taken helps to control Diabetes.

6. Chewing few leaves of Sweet Neem (Curry patta) everyday morning also helps to reduce Diabetes.

7. Eating an Indian gooseberry (Amla) everyday helps in reducing Diabetes.

8. Dip Fenugreek (Menthi) seeds overnight, eat them in the empty stomach in the morning or use fresh Fenugreek leaves in cooking which cures Diabetes.

9. Indian gooseberry (Amla) powder with Turmeric powder taken in the empty stomach also helps to reduce Diabetes.

10. Drinking Lemon water in the morning helps in reducing Diabetes.

11. Beal fruit taken in any form is also helpful in reducing Diabetes.

12. Salted Buttermilk (Chach) taken in the morning helps to reduce Diabetes.

13. Nut Meg (Jay phal) powder with pure Ghee taken regularly helps to reduce Diabetes.

14. Orange skin dried in the shade and powdered. A spoon of this powder boiled in water and filtered, this decoction taken helps to reduce Diabetes.

15. Eating Tomato juice or raw Tomato regularly helps to reduce Diabetes.

16. Basil leaves (Tulsi) chewed in the morning helps in reducing Diabetes.

17. Sadabahar (Vinka rosia) is good to reduce the blood sugar level. Boil one glass of water in half glass of water, Put 3 flowers of Sadabahar, leave for 5 minutes then drink the water by removing the flower. Then drink the other half glass of hot water. Continue for 7 days which is a good remedy for curing Diabetes.

Chapter 20

Diarrhoea

Loose and inconsistent stools are indications of diarrhoea, diarrhoea is an effective way for the body to get rid of an undesirable substance and this may be followed with symptoms like vomiting, stomach pain, thirst, fever, nausea, dehydration. But it can be dangerous especially for children and old aged people if not treated immediately. Sometimes stool in diarrheoa contains blood also.

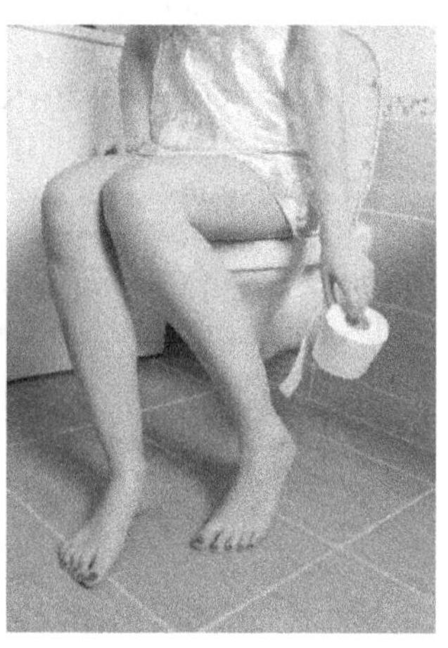

Diarrhoea may be due to food poisoning, bacterial infection due to the use of contaminated food or water, food allergies, excessive use of alcohol or laxatives or spicy food or caffeine, improper and insufficient sleep, constipation, side effects of allopathic medicines.

Human body uses diarrhea to flush out bacteria or viruses which might have ingested by eating contaminated food. So it might not be advisable to stop diarrhea too quickly. However, if diarrhea goes on for several days, dehydration and loss of important nutrients may occur which can be fatal especially in children. It may lead to gastritis, enteritis, gastroenteritis etc. Diarrhea can be stopped with medication, but the medicines may interfere with the natural process of cleansing, that the body desperately needs. With natural remedies we may help ourselves feel better without stopping the immune system from its work. So we can use the natural home made remedies to cure diarrheoa.

Remedies for Diarrheoa

1. A glass of water can be boiled and cooled. Slight sugar and salt can be added. Drinking this water frequently helps to avoid dehydration during Diarrhoea.
2. Drinking Lemon juice 4-5 times a day helps to cure Diarrhoea.
3. Pomegranate (Anar) leaves boiled in water with Sugar and filtered. Drinking this decoction 3 times a day helps to cure Diarrhoea.
4. Drinking half cup of Mint (Pudina) juice in every two hours helps to cure Diarrhoea.
5. Wall nut (Akhroat) grinded with water and this paste applied on the naval helps to cure Diarrhoea.
6. Drinking Basil (Tulsi) juice mixed with Betel (Pan) juice helps to cure Diarrhoea.
7. Orange juice mixed with Milk taken helps to cure Diarrhoea especially for children.
8. Eating a spoon of Dhania (Coriander) powder with Black salt after meals is helpful in curing Diarrhoea.
9. Drinking hot water mixed with Ginger juice once in an hour helps to cure Diarrhoea.
10. A spoon of pure Ghee (made from cows milk or buffaloes milk) taken with hot water both morning and evening helps to cure Diarrhoea.
11. Eating a spoon of Carrom seeds (Ajwain) powder with hot water helps to reduce Diarrhoea.
12. Eating a ripe Banana with Buttermilk (Chach) is a good remedy to cure Diarrhoea.
13. Apple pieces without skin boiled in milk taken 3 times a day (but not directly Apple juice) cures Diarrhoea.
14. One gram of Neem seeds and one gram of Sugar taken with hot water and eating only boiled Rice with Curd in the meals cures Diarrhoea.
15. Eating Carrot is good for curing prolonged Diarrhoea.
16. One spoon of Ginger juice, half cup of Curd mixed with half cup of Mango juice and taken helps to cure Diarrhoea.

17. For watery Diarrhoea, taking a spoon of roasted Cumin seeds (Jeera) with half spoon of Honey 4 times a day is helpful.

18. For watery Diarrhoea taking roasted Cumin seeds (Jeera) and Black salt with Buttermilk after meals is helpful.

19. Boil Aniseed (Sauf) with water and filtered. This filtered water can be used to make wheat flour dough for making Rotis. eating these Rotis are beneficial during Diarrhoea.

20. Taking two teaspoon of Flea seeds (Isabgol) with Curd both in the morning and evening cures Diarrhoea.

21. 2 grams of Cinnamon (Dalchini) powder taken with warm water 3 times a day helps to cure Diarrhoea.

22. For Diarrhoea in children it is advisable to give Aniseeds (Sauf) water with a pinch of Black salt.

23. A spoon of Honey taken with half glass of Buttermilk (Chach) helps to cure Diarrhoea.

24. Mix few Flea seeds (Isabgol) with Curd. Add Salt, dry Ginger (Saunth), Cumin seeds (Jeera) powder and drinking this for few days helps to cure Diarrhoea.

25. Eating Lentil (Masoor dal) is good for people having Diarrhoea.

26. Onion paste applied on the naval helps to stop Diarrhoea.

27. Half spoon of Dry Gooseberries (Amla) powder mixed with same quantity of Black salt taken with water helps to cure Diarrhoea.

28. Eating boiled raw Papaya (Papita) is good for Diarrhoea.

29. Boil tender Guava (Amrud) leaves with water, filtered and drinking this decoction helps to cure Diarrhoea.

30. Left out water after boiling Rice (Chawal) is good for Diarrhoea. For children half cup and for adults one cup of this water can be given which cures Diarrhoea.

31. Taking Half cup of Mango juice and 25 gm Curd with a spoon of Ginger helps to cure prolonged Diarrhoea.

32. Take 3 Black berry (Jamun) leaves, neither too tender nor too ripe, grind them with Rock salt (Saindha namak) and

make a tablet of it and take one tablet both morning and evening to get instant cure for Diarrhoea.

Remedies for Blood in Stool During Diarrhoea.

1. Taking Mango seed powder with Buttermilk is a good remedy to cure Diarrhoea.
2. Fenugreek (Menthi) seeds powder taken with Buttermilk or Curd helps to stop Diarrhoea.
3. 20 grams of Black berry (Jamun) seeds grinded with water and taken twice a day helps to stop Diarrhoea.
4. Drinking half spoon of Lemon juice with Goat milk helps to stop Diarrhoea.
5. Onion pieces or Spring onion (Onion flower) taken with fresh Curd also stops Diarrhoea.
6. Pomegranate juice (Anar) taken 3 times a day gives relief from Diarrhoea.
7. Drinking Pomegranate juice (Anar) mixed with equal quantity of Sugarcane (Ganna) juice helps to cure Diarrhoea.
8. 15 gram of Coriander powder (Dhania) and 12 grams of Sugar candy (Mishri) taken with water stops Diarrhoea.
9. Taking Ber Fruit (Zizyphus) helps to cure wounds in the intestine during Diarrhoea.
10. Sweet Neem (Curry patta) leaves grinded and taken with Buttermilk or chewing Sweet Neem leaves with pure Honey stops Diarrhoea.
11. Eating Dates (Khajur) everyday helps to overcome loss of nutrients during Diarrhoea.
12. Pomegranate (Anar) skin grinded and taken with Buttermilk stops Diarrhoea.
13. Making Tea with Cardamom powder (Elaichi) and drinking this tea also stops Diarrhoea.
14. Eating Banana with Sugar or eating Banana mixed with Buttermilk also cures Diarrhoea.
15. Chewing Carrom (Ajwain) seeds after every meal also stops Diarrhoea.

16. Eating Boiled Jo (Barley) also helps to stop Diarrhoea.
17. Beet root juice mixed with Honey can be taken which helps to stop Diarrhoea.
18. Mix Guava (Amrud) pulp without seeds and a spoon of Honey in Milk. Drinking this milk helps in curing Diarrhoea.
19. Eating small pieces of raw Mango or grounded raw Mango skin with Buttermilk twice a day also helps in curing Diarrhoea.
20. Taking Banana pulp and Tamarind (Imli) pulp mixed in a glass of Buttermilk for 2-3 days cures Diarrhoea.

Dry and Chapped Lips

Dry and chapped lips can be because of many reasons. In winter, this problem is common. Other than that when you are having cold, fever you will feel your lips are dried up as you are breathing thru mouth. There are some home remedies for this dry and chopped lips problem.

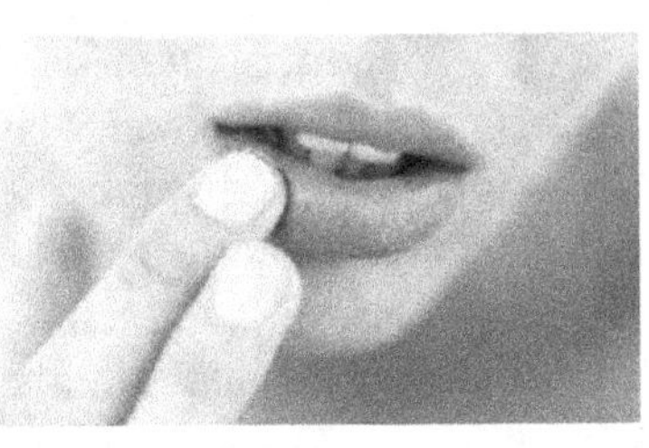

Remedies for Dry and Chapped Lips

1. Applying 2 -3 drops of Mustard (Sarson) oil in the naval after bath and before going to bed is the best remedy for curing dry and chapped lips problem.

2. Applying pure Ghee or pure Butter or Coconut oil on the lips cures dry and chapped lips problem.

3. Applying Glycerin on the lips also helps to overcome dry and chapped lips problem.

4. Pure Butter mixed with a pinch of Salt applied on the lips cures dry and chapped lips problem.

5. Eating Almonds (Badam) everyday helps to overcome dry and chapped lips problem.

6. Cardamom (Elaichi) powder mixed with Butter can be taken for 7 days will completely cure dry and chapped lips problem.

7. Rub a fresh Aloe Vera (Gwar Patha) leaf on the lips which helps to overcome dry and chapped lips problem.

8. Applying fresh Milk cream on the lips helps to cure dry and chapped lips problem.

Chapter 22

Dry Cough

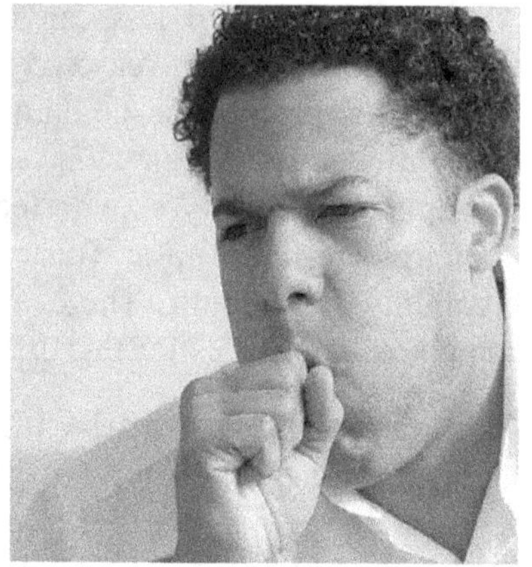

A Dry Cough is often known as unproductive cough as it does not include any mucus. It usually occurs due to excessive dust in the air, smoking, climatic changes, pollen and allergens. Cough is a natural defense mechanism of the human body to clear the throat of any type of blockages so that breathing becomes easy and possible.

There are many home remedies to treat dry cough. Most of these remedies prove to be effective but the results may vary from one person to another.

Remedies for Dry Cough

1. Glycyrriza glabra (Jyeshta madhu) powder mixed with Lemon juice and Honey taken thrice a day cures Dry cough.
2. Taking Jaggery (Gur) mixed with few drops of Mustard (Sarson) oil helps to cure Dry cough.
3. Eating Dates (Khajur) also helps to cures Dry cough.
4. Drinking Sugar cane (Ganna) juice also helps to get relief from Dry cough.
5. Black pepper (Kali mirch) and Sugar candy (Mishri) powdered and mixed with pure Ghee can be made like a ball, sucked slowly to get relief from Dry cough.

6. Almonds (Badam) and Black pepper (Kali mirch) crushed and boiled with Milk for 10 minutes later added with red Sugar candy (Mishri) or Sugar and taken hot without filtering cures Dry cough.

7. Ginger paste cooked with Jaggery (Gur) and small quantity of Ghee can be made into small balls. Sucking this ball gives instant relief and cures Dry cough.

Chapter 23

Excessive Sweating

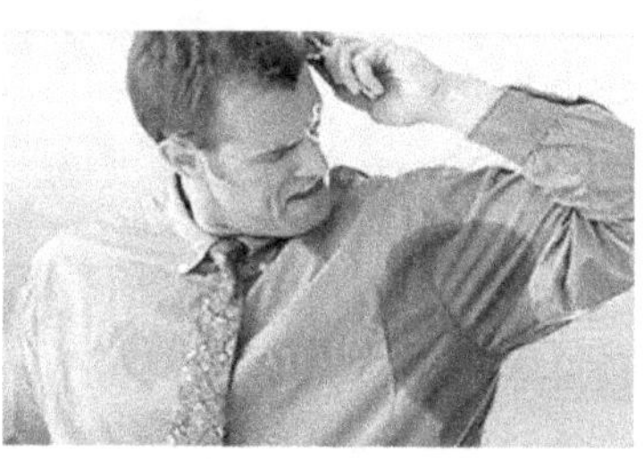

Sweat is body's natural mechanism for waste disposal and temperature control. Some people sweat more than others-in a condition called Hyperhydrosis. The most vulnerable areas are armpits, groin and feet.

Remedies for Excessive Sweating

1. Harad (Haritaki) grinded and applied on the body 10 minutes before bath helps to cure excessive sweating problem.
2. Goose berry (Amla) juice applied on the affected area before bath cures excessive sweating problem.
3. Raw Brinjal (Byangan) paste applied on the affected area before bath cures excessive sweating problem.
4. Alum (Phitkari) dissolved in water can be used to wash the affected parts which helps to cure excessive sweating problem.
5. Brinjal pieces with Poppy seeds (Khus Khus) grinded and this paste applied on the affected area before bath cures excessive sweating problem.
6. Roasted Green gram (Moong) powder mixed with water to make a paste. This paste rubbed on the affected area before bath helps to cure excessive sweating problem.
7. Brinjal pieces dipped in water for sometime and this water used to wash the affected parts cures excessive sweating problem.

Chapter 24

Gas/Flatulence

Causes of this are improper digestive system, wrong food habits, constipation, eating without chewing, eating and drinking simultaneously, too much fried and spicy foods, non vegetarian foods etc.

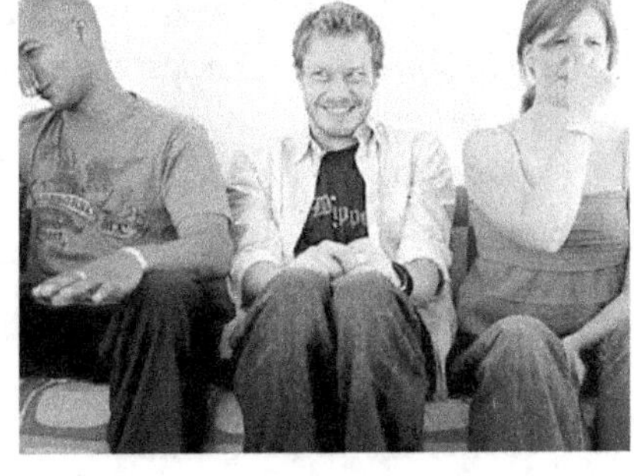

Avoid gas forming eatables like Capsicum (Shimla mirch), Maida, fried items, Pigeon pea (Arhar dal), Black gram (Urad) etc. and also avoid heavy foods which are difficult to digest.

Remedies for Gas/Flatulence

1. Eating Carrom (Ajwain) seeds and Black salt with hot water gives immediate relief from gas or flatulence.
2. Eating a piece of Jaggery (Gur) after every meals helps to get relief from gas or flatulence.
3. Eating Orange in the morning cleans the intestine thereby reducing gas formation or eating Orange with Black salt gives instant relief from gas or flatulence.
4. Eating Radish (Muli) with Salt and Back pepper (Kali mirch) helps to overcome gas or flatulence. But remember Radish digests everything but it cannot digest itself so after eating Radish eat a piece of Jaggery or eat Radish leaves.
5. Drinking Mint (Pudina) juice helps to get instant relief from gas or flatulence.

6. Eating Turmeric and Salt with water also gives instant relief from gas or flatulence.

7. Guava (Amrud) taken with Salt everyday morning helps to overcome gas or flatulence problem.

8. Sprouted Fenugreek (Menthi) seeds or Fenugreek seeds taken with salted Buttermilk (Chach) helps to get relief from gas or flatulence.

9. Chewing a piece of Ginger before meals improves digestion and helps in reducing gas formation.

10. Using Asafoetida (Hing), Fenugreek (Menthi) seeds, Cumin seeds (Jeera), Carrom seeds (Ajwain), Garlic, Ginger regularly in cooking helps to overcome gas or flatulence problem.

11. Drinking Bitter gourd juice (Karela) helps to overcome gas, flatulence problem.

12. Boil 5-6 Cloves (Laung) in water. Drink this after cooling which helps to overcome gas or flatulence.

13. Asafoetida (Hing) paste applied on the naval gives instant relief from gas or flatulence.

14. Taking roasted Cumin (Jeera) powder with Honey after meals helps to reduce gas or flatulence problem.

15. Lemon juice and Black pepper (Kali mirch) powder taken with Hot water helps to overcome gas or flatulence.

16. Boil Ginger piece or Long pepper (Pipple) or Black pepper (Kali mirch) powder or Cumin seeds (Jeera) in Milk helps to overcome gas or flatulence problem due to plain milk.

17. Drinking Cabbage (Patta gobi) juice or Carrot juice helps to overcome gas or flatulence.

18. Sitting 5 minutes in a upright posture (Vajrasan) after every meals gives instant and permanent relief from gas or flatulence.

19. Raw Garlic taken regularly or using Garlic in cooking helps to overcome gas problem.

Chapter 25

Giddiness/Dizziness

Giddiness is a whirling sensation in which you feel like falling. Giddiness can be because of many reasons like weakness, anemia, head aches, fever, pitta, heat, gastric etc .The main solution is to solve the root problem .Here we have given some home remedies for instant relief.

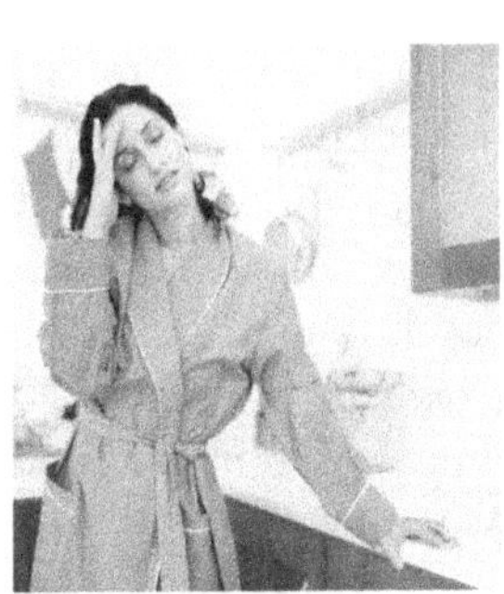

Remedies for Giddiness/Dizziness

1. Drinking a cup of hot water with two spoons of Lemon juice gives instant relief from Giddiness.
2. Drinking water mixed with Lemon juice, Jaggery (Gur) or Sugar, Cardamom powder (Elaichi) gives instant relief from Giddiness.
3. Drinking Basil (Tulsi) juice mixed with Sugar helps to get relief from Giddiness problem.
4. Coriander (Dhania) seeds boiled in water with Sugar candy (Mishri), filtered and drinking this decoction give instant relief from Giddiness.
5. Two spoons of Carrom leaves (Ajwain) juice taken everyday helps to overcome Giddiness problem.
6. Taking Pineapple pieces with Salt gives instant relief from Giddiness.
7. Eating Gooseberry (Amla) with Sugar or eating its Morabba also helps to control Giddiness.

Chapter 26

Grey Hair

Premature Graying of hair is a common problem now a days. It can be because of chemical pollution in air and water, Use of shampoos, conditioners, hair driers, synthetic hair products, packed foods etc. Other than this our body factors like decreased Melanin pigment, too much of anger, 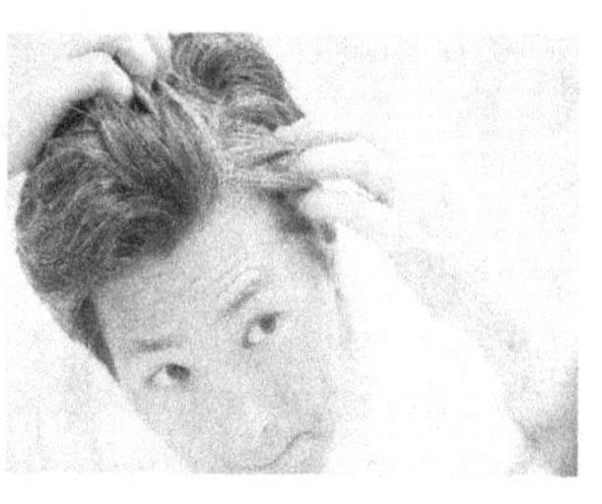 depression, mental tension, sadness, cold, continuous exposure to hot sun, hereditary factors, hormonal imbalance, constipation, excessive coffee, tea, chocolate, alcohol consumption etc.

Remedies for Grey Hair

1. Applying Onion paste on the scalp for few days before taking bath helps grey hair to turn black gradually.
2. Lemon juice mixed with Gooseberry (Amla) powder applied on the scalp for few days helps grey hair to turn black gradually.
3. Eating Sesame (Til) seeds daily and applying its oil regularly helps grey hair to turn black.
4. Eating Fenugreek (Menthi) sprouts regularly and applying Fenugreek paste on the scalp an hour before taking bath once in a week helps to overcome grey hair problem..
5. Bael leaves grinded and applied 2 hours before taking bath regularly helps to overcome grey hair problem.
6. Durva (Dub, a grass used to worship Lord Ganesha) paste applied before taking bath regularly helps grey hair to turn black gradually.

7. Regularly applying Butter or Butter mixed with Fenugreek powder on the scalp and taking bath with cold water helps to overcome grey hair problem.

8. Half cup of Curd Mixed with a pinch of Black pepper (Kali mirch) powder and a spoon of Lemon juice applied 15 minutes before taking bath helps grey hair to turn black slowly.

9. Regular application of Henna (Mehandi) paste applied an hour before taking bath helps grey hair to turn black slowly.

10. Drinking Wheat grass juice everyday helps to overcome grey hair problem.

11. Boil Triphala (Triphala is composed of Harad (Haritaki), Amla (Indian gooseberries) and Behada (Bibhitaki) powder in Gingery (Thil) oil and this filtered oil applied regularly on the scalp helps grey hair to turn black .

12. Guava (Amrud) leaves grinded and applied regularly on the hair before taking bath helps grey hair to turn black slowly.

13. Neem seeds grinded and applied on the scalp and boiled Neem leaves used for washing hair helps grey hair to turn black slowly.

14. Massaging scalp regularly with Ghee (Prepared from cow milk) also helps to overcome grey hair problem.

15. Drinking Carrot juice everyday helps to keep hair black and helps to overcome grey hair problem.

Hair Fall

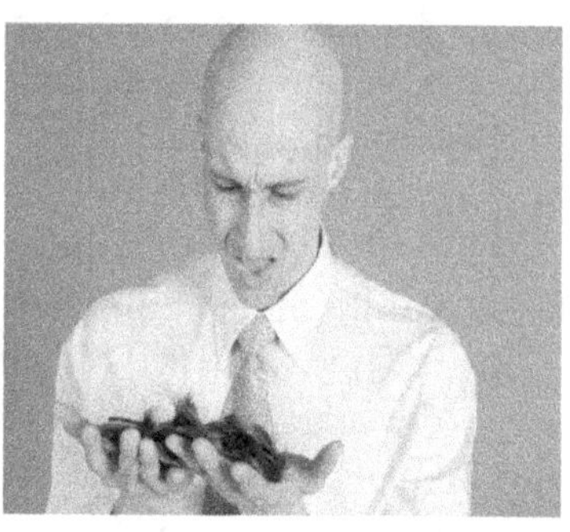

Hair fall (50 to 100 strands per day) is normal but excessive hair fall can be because of many reasons like dandruff, Anemia, prolonged fever, nutritional deficiency, stress, medications, toxins in food and water, Typhoid, hair lice, uncleanness, lack of use of hair oil, hormonal changes, Very hot weather, using too much of cosmetics like soap, shampoo, hair colours, hair driers, etc.

Prevention

1. Take regular head bath to keep the hairs clean. Until necessary don't use hot water which harms the hair roots.

2. Regular combing increases blood circulation in the scalp which strengthens the hair roots.

3. Instead of soap, shampoo, conditioners, hair driers go for natural hair cleansing products.

4. Massage hair roots with oil regularly. You can make your own hair oil as mentioned below.

5. Dandruff causes hair fall so it should be treated immediately.

6. Eat healthy diet with lots of fruits and vegetables. Avoid coffee, tea, smoking etc which harms the hair roots.

Remedies for Hair Fall

1. Fenugreek (Menthi) paste applied regularly on the scalp an hour before taking bath helps to overcome hair fall problem.

2. Hibiscus leaves boiled in small quantity of water and used along with Shikakai as a hair wash instead of soap, shampoo helps in controlling hair fall problem. This is also a natural hair conditioner.

3. Neem paste applied regularly on the scalp before taking bath also reduces hair fall problem.

4. Durva (Dub, a grass used to worship Lord Ganesha) paste applied regularly on the scalp before taking bath helps to control hair fall.

5. Fenugreek paste mixed with Castor oil (Erand) applied regularly before taking bath helps to overcome hair fall problem.

6. Betel leaves (Pan) grinded and mixed with Gingery (Til) oil or Betel leaves (Pan) grinded and mixed with Coconut oil applied on the scalp before taking bath helps to overcome hair fall problem.

7. Eating Gooseberry (Amla) everyday and applying Gooseberry paste on the scalp regularly before taking bath helps to control hair fall.

8. Applying Lemon juice on the scalp 10 minutes before taking bath helps to control hair fall problem.

9. Soap nut powder used as a hair wash or soap nut leaves paste applied on the scalp before taking bath helps to reduce hair fall problem.

10. Henna paste (Mehandi) mixed with yellow portion of egg or Henna paste with Lemon juice applied on the scalp regularly before taking bath helps to reduce hair fall.

11. Beet root leaves grinded with Henna leaves applied regularly on the scalp before taking bath helps to reduce hair fall problem.

12. Drinking Wheat grass juice every morning for one and half month cures hair fall problem.

13. Basil (Tulsi) paste mixed with Gooseberry (Amla) powder applied 10 minutes before taking bath helps to control hair fall problem.

14. Tea powder boiled in water can be used as a hair wash, which helps in reducing hair fall problem.

15. Eating Amaranth (Cholayi), Cabbage (Patta gobi) regularly helps to overcome hair fall problem.

16. You can make a hair oil of your own like this. Boil Fenugreek(Menthi) seeds, Neem or Sweet Neem (Curry patta) leaves, Gooseberry (Amla), Henna leaves (Mehandi), some Basil (Tulsi) leaves, in Coconut oil or Gingery oil for 20 minutes in slow flame and store it. Use this regularly to overcome all hair related problems.

17. Gram flour (Besan) mixed with Curd or Gram flour mixed with Milk used as a hair wash helps to overcome hair fall problem.

18. Applying crushed raw Papaya (Papita) paste on the scalp 10 minutes before taking bath is very helpful. This process assists in the exfoliation of dandruff flakes and slows down fungal growth. Papaya contains enzyme Papain which is very helpful in controlling hair fall.

Chapter 28

Head Ache

There can be many reasons for head ache like cold, sinus problems, mental tensions, stomach problems, indigestion, heat, migrane, high blood pressure, fever, inadequate sleep, eye problems, allergies, gastric, constipation, brain problems and many more reasons. Sometimes it is difficult to know the reason for a head ache, like in case 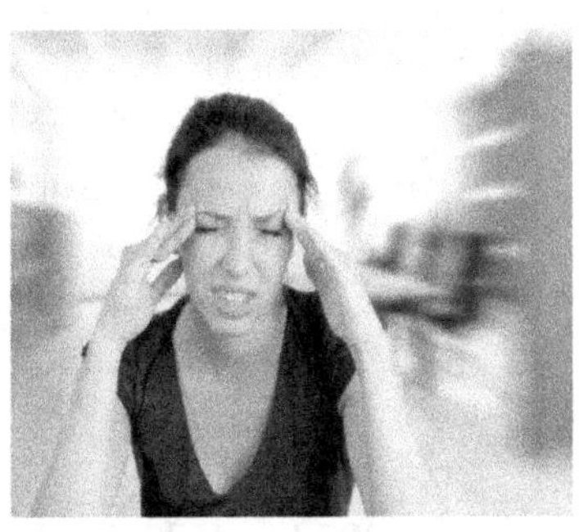 of migrane. But in general if we know the reason of headache it can be treated accordingly. It is always advisable to keep the stomach clean, sleep properly, avoid unnecessary tensions and treat for cold, constipation, eye sight problems if required.

Remedies for Head Ache

1. Taking Steam containing Eucalyptus oil drops or decongestant vaporizing ointments like Vicks vaporub, Sensur or only steam helps to get rid of headache due to cold congestion or sinus problems.
2. Applying Eucalyptus oil on the forehead also helps to relieve headache due to cold.
3. Equal quantities of Cumin seeds (Jeera), Black pepper (Kali mirch), Coriander seeds (Dhania), Dry ginger (Saunth) powdered. A spoon of this powder boiled in water with Jaggery (Gur) and taken before sleep helps to get relief from head ache due to cold.

4. Eating an Apple everyday with salt helps to overcome headache.

5. Cinnamon (Dalchini) grinded with Lemon juice applied on the forehead helps to get relief from head ache.

6. Dry Coconut chewed with Sugar candy (Mishri) helps to get relief from headache.

7. Applying Castor oil (Erand ka teil) or Gingery oil (Til oil) or Coconut oil (Narial) on the centre of the head helps to get relief from head ache.

8. Tamarind (Imli) mixed in water with Jaggery (Gur), filtered and taken twice a day helps to overcome headache which comes because of heat.

9. Applying Garlic paste on the forehead relives headache but not to be rubbed as it can cause irritation and burning of the skin. Some people's skin is more sensitive so in case of any discomfort this remedy can be avoided.

10. Eating Jo (Barley) regularly helps to overcome headache problem.

11. A spoon of tender Neem leaf juice taken everyday helps to overcome headache.

12. Pomegranate (Anar) juice with Honey taken for a week helps to get relief from head ache due to mental tensions.

13. Black pepper grinded with Drumstick (Muranka bhaji) leaves applied on the forehead helps to get relief from headache.

14. Taking Lemon Tea helps to get relief from headache due to Pitta problem.

15. Applying Ginger paste on the forehead and sleeping covering the body with a blanket helps to get relief from head ache.

16. Taking raw Onion or smelling Onion juice will help to get relief from head ache.

17. Black gram (Urad) grinded and applied on the forehead helps to get relief from head ache.

18. Putting pure Ghee (made from cow's milk) drops in both the nostrils regularly helps to cure head ache permanently.

19. Massaging foot soles with Ghee or Mustard (Sarson) oil in the nights regularly helps to cure head ache.

20. Boil some Cloves (Laung) with Jaggery (Gur) in water for few minutes, filter it and take this decoction twice a day or just applying Clove paste on the forehead helps to get relief from headache.

21. Applying diluted Asafoetida (Hing) paste on the forehead gives relief from headache but be careful as it can cause irritation and burn the skin.

22. Applying Mint juice (Pudina) on the fore head helps to get relief from headache.

23. Cardamom (Elaichi) paste applied on the forehead or smelling Cardamom helps to get relief from head ache.

24. Drinking Water melon juice or Bael juice helps to relieve from headache due to heat.

25. Drinking Basil (Tulsi) juice mixed with Lemon juice helps to get relief from head ache.

26. Drinking Coffee also helps sometimes to get relief from head ache.

27. Having Lemon juice with Cardamom (Elaichi) powder helps to get relief from headache.

Chapter 29

Head Lice

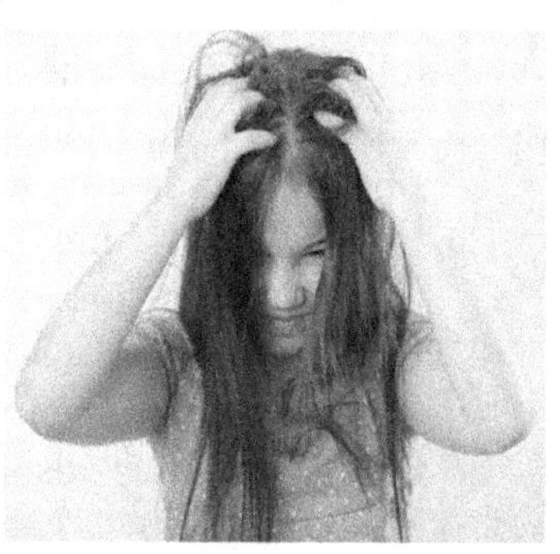

Head Lice's are highly contagious and it is extremely important that they should be eliminated as quickly and completely as possible as they will start weakening the roots of hairs and causes itching, hair fall etc. Some home remedies have given which can be applied to solve hair lice problem.

Remedies for Head Lice

1. Guava (Amrud) leaves grinded and mixed with Turmeric applied on the scalp 2 hrs before taking bath helps in getting rid of head lice.

2. Neem leaves grinded and applied on the scalp 2 hours before taking bath helps in getting rid of head lice.

3. Half spoon of Black pepper (Kali mirch) powder and one cup Curd mixed with two spoons of Lemon juice applied on the scalp 20 minutes before taking bath destroys head lice completely but remember to close eyes while taking bath as Black pepper can cause irritation to the eyes.

4. Rubbing a Lemon piece on the scalp or applying Lemon juice with Coconut oil before taking bath helps to destroy head lice completely.

5. Beet root leaves boiled and squeezed and this squeezed water applied on the scalp before taking bath destroys head lice.

6. Rubbing boiled White goose foot (Bathua leaves) on the scalp 20 minutes before taking bath destroys head lice.
7. Garlic kills lices as it is pungent. Garlic paste mixed with Lemon juice applied on the scalp before taking bath destroys head lice.
8. Basil (Tulsi) leaves grinded with Neem leaves applied on the scalp before taking bath destroys head lice.
9. Putting Neem leaves and Basil leaves under the pillow helps to overcome hair lice problem.
10. You can make your own hair oil like this: Boil Neem leaves, Basil leaves, Gooseberry (Amla), Cloves (Laung), in Coconut oil and this can be used regularly to avoid all hair related problems.

Chapter 30

Hiccough

Though Hiccough is common and a minor thing, prolonged Hiccough can be a indication of diseases like epilepsy, hysteria, kidney diseases, tumors, etc. Minor Hiccough can be due to eating very quickly, taking a cold drink while eating hot food, eating very hot or spicy food, laughing vigorously or coughing, or drinking excessive alcohol etc.

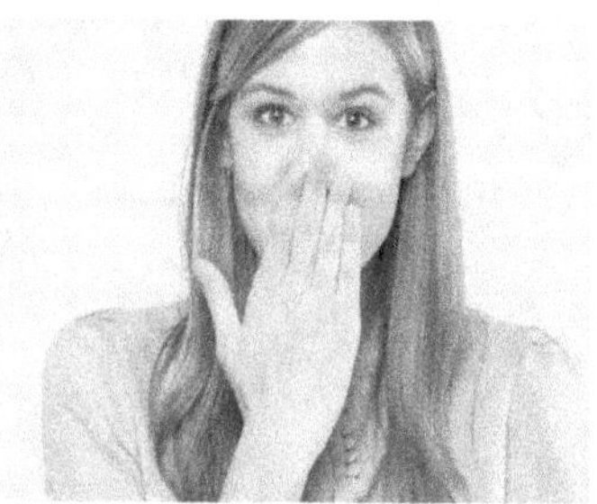

Remedies for Hiccough

1. Holding breath as much as possible stops Hiccough.
2. Diverting attention stops Hiccough.
3. If Hiccough is due to indigestion then taking water with soda helps. Remember not to drink anything hot.
4. Sucking Sugar or Jaggery (Gur) or Sugar candy (Mishri) or Ginger or Clove helps to stop Hiccough.
5. Chewing Radish (Muli) leaves gives instant relief from Hiccough.
6. Chewing Mint (Pudina) leaves gives instant relief from Hiccough
7. Sucking Lemon piece gives instant relief from Hiccough.
8. Dry Ginger powder smelled also stops Hiccough.
9. Eating a spoon of Honey gives instant relief from Hiccough.
10. Drinking Sugar cane (Ganna) juice helps to overcome Hiccough.

11. Drinking a spoon of Basil juice (Tulsi) with half spoon of Honey twice a day helps to stop prolonged and regular Hiccough.

12. Eating a pinch of Asafoetida (Hing) kept inside a Banana fruit pulp or Asafoetida with Jaggery helps to stop Hiccough immediately.

13. Onion piece taken with Salt stops hiccough. Repeat every hour till Hiccough stops.

14. Chewing a piece of Cinnamon (Dalchini) also stops Hiccough within a moment.

15. Chewing Cardamoms (Elaichi) also stops Hiccough immediately.

16. Steam of water mixed with Black pepper powder helps to stop Hiccough.

17. Taking 2 spoons of Ginger juice with 100 milliliter of Milk helps to stop Hiccough.

8. A spoon of Pure Ghee heated and taken hot also stops Hiccough.

19. In 20 milliliter of Neem juice, add one fourth spoon of Long pepper (Pipple) powder with one spoon of Honey and this can be taken 3-4 times a day to cure prolonged and regular Hiccough.

20. Banyan fruits taken with Honey cures Hiccough.

20. Mix dry Ginger (Saunth) with Jaggery (Gur) powder and make small balls like a pea nut and sucking this helps to stop Hiccough.

21. Equal quantity of Long pepper (Pipple) and Dhania (Coriander) powdered. Taking 3 grams of this with a spoon of Honey twice a day helps to cure prolonged and regular Hiccough.

22. Taking a spoon of Lemon juice and a spoon of Honey mixed with a pinch of Black salt stops hiccough. Repeat every 20 minutes till Hiccough stops.

23. Dry Gooseberry (Amla), dry Ginger (Saunth), Long pepper (Pipple) and Sugar candy (Mishri) all this powdered together and taking 3 grams of this mixture in every two hours helps to stop prolonged and regular Hiccough.
24. Peacock feather can be burnt and smelled stops severe Hiccough.
25. Dry Banana leaf can be burnt and smelled can stop severe Hiccough.

31. High Blood Pressure

Hypertension is generally defined as a blood pressure greater than 140/90. Elevated blood pressure raises your risk for heart attack, stroke, brain hammerages etc.

Remedies for High Blood Pressure

1. Keeping stomach clean, Reducing Salt intake and adequate sleep helps to control high blood pressure.
2. Eating Papaya (Papita) everyday morning helps to control high blood pressure.
3. Sweet Neem (Curry patta) used regularly in cooking and drinking Sweet Neem juice helps to control high blood pressure.
4. Eating Beetroot everyday with Lemon juice helps to control high blood pressure.
5. Drinking Bottle gourd juice (Ghea) everyday helps to control high blood pressure.
6. Watermelon helps in controlling high blood pressure. Watermelon seeds helps to widen the capillaries which makes high blood pressure to come down. The seeds powdered and boiled in water, filtered and this decoction taken helps to control high blood pressure.
7. Regular body massage helps to control high blood pressure.

8. Half cup of Banana stem juice taken twice a day helps to control high blood pressure.

9. Lemon juice helps to make capillaries flexible. Drinking hot water with Lemon juice in the morning helps to overcome high blood pressure problem.

10. Store water in a cleaned Copper jug overnight and drink a glass of this water in the morning helps to control high blood pressure.

12. Boiled Joe (Barley) taken with Buttermilk (Chach) and Lemon juice regularly helps to control high blood pressure.

13. Chewing a raw Garlic everyday in empty stomach with a spoon of Honey helps to control high blood pressure problem.

14. Tinda (Tinda Pharsi) helps to increase urine formation and helps to control high blood pressure.

15. Eating Apple regularly helps to control high blood pressure.

16. Drinking Ash Gourd (Petha) juice everyday in the empty stomach helps to control high blood pressure.

17. Colcasia (Arbi) also helps high blood pressure to come down.

18. Honey taken regularly helps to make the capillaries active and reduces high blood pressure.

19. Mint (Pudina) juice taken regularly helps to maintain the blood pressure.

20. Boiled Potato helps to reduce high blood pressure as it contains magnesium in it.

21. Eating Amaranth (Cholayi) in any form helps to control high blood pressure.

22. Drinking Tomato juice or eating Tomato regularly in the morning helps to control high blood pressure.

23. Two spoons of Carrot juice taken with a spoon of Spinach (Palak) juice regularly helps to control high blood pressure.

24. Eating Goose berries (Amla) everyday or eating its Morabba helps to control high blood pressure.
25. Taking a spoon of Triphala (Triphala is composed of Harad (Terminalia chebula, Haritaki), Indian gooseberries (Amla) and Behada (Bibhitaki)) every day helps to control high blood pressure.
26. Putting Henna (Mehandi) paste on the head or foot sole which extracts the body heat and control high blood pressure.

Chapter 32

Improve Appetite

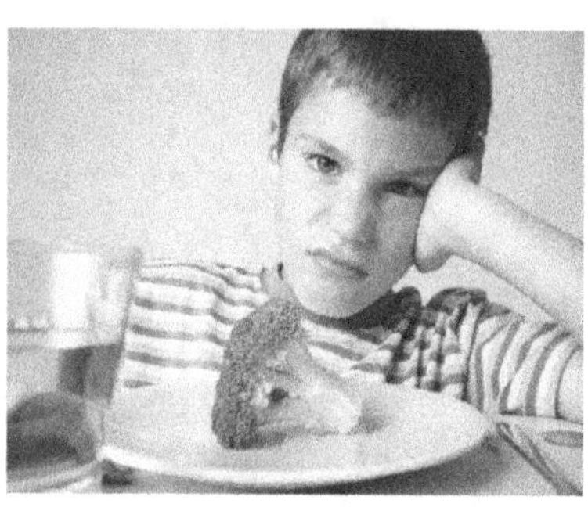

Reluctance to consume food or loss of appetite can be caused by many and different factors both physiological and mental. People who are much stressed or are going through emotional turmoil are extremely sensible and can develop loss of appetite. Prolonged suffering from a severe disease, gastrointestinal disorders or some medications can also lead to this disorder. The tendency of snacking or overeating between meals leads to different liver problems and then to loss of appetite.

The consumption of large quantities of non alcoholic and alcoholic drinks is another factor for this disorder. There are people that refuse to eat because they are afraid they will get fat. They adopt very severe diets and deprive their body of essential nutrients. In this case we confront with anorexia, a more severe disorder. It usually hampers the normal functions of the vital organs and can cause even the death of the person who suffers from anorexia.

Loss of appetite can be easily treated. It is very important not to neglect it because secondary complication might appear if the immunity decreases under its normal level.

Remedies for Improve Appetite

1. Eating Black berries (Jamun) regularly, helps in improving Appetite.

2. Drinking Coriander (Dhania) juice mixed with water regularly helps in improving Appetite.
3. Taking Carrom seeds (Ajwain) and Black salt with hot water, helps in improving Appetite.
4. Californian Raisin (Monakka), Salt, Black pepper (Kali Mirch) taken together with hot water, helps to improve Appetite.
5. Eating a piece of Ginger before meals, helps in improving Appetite.
6. Eating Raw Cucumber (Kheera), Raw radish (Muli), Raw white Onion, all are helpful in improving Appetite.
7. Eating Tomato, Amaranth (Red Cholayi), Bitter gourd (Karela), Fenugreek (Menthi) regularly, helps in improving Appetite.
8. Drinking Tamarind (Imli) water mixed with Salt and Black pepper (Kali mirch), helps in improving Appetite.
9. Eating Ber (Zizyphus) fruit regularly helps in improving Appetite.
10. Eating Orange with Black salt helps in improving Appetite.
11. Drinking sour tasted Apple juice with Sugar Candy (Mishri) for few days helps to improve Appetite.
12. Sugar cane (Ganna) juice with Honey, Lemon juice and a pinch of Clove (Laung) powder taken together, helps to improve Appetite.
13. Sweet Neem (Curry patta), Garlic can be used regularly in cooking, which helps to improve Appetite.
14. Lemon juice mixed with Ginger juice and Salt taken with water helps to improve Appetite.

Chapter 33

Increase Weight

Some people who are under weight can follow these home remedies to increase their weight.

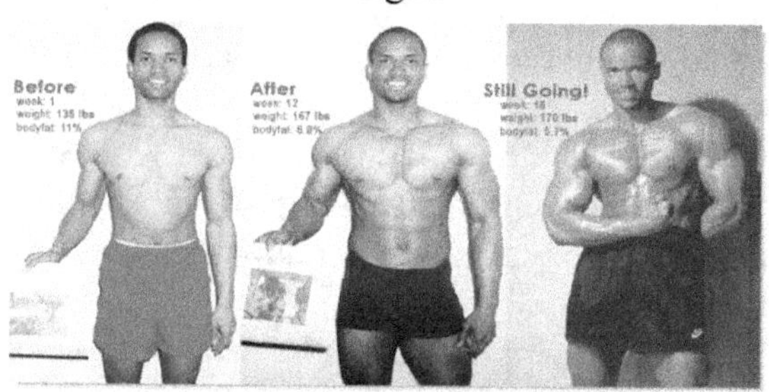

Remedies to Increase Weight

1. Eating Cashew nut (Kaju) regularly or eating its sweet will increase weight but avoid its overeating.
2. Ripe Banana pulp meshed with Milk and Sugar or a Banana with Milk can be taken regularly which helps to increase weight.
3. Drinking Mango milk shake helps to increase weight.
4. Drinking Goat milk regularly also helps to increase weight.
5. Banana flower grinded and this juice taken with Milk also helps to increase weight.
6. Jo (Barley) without skin boiled with Milk and Sugar can be taken everyday helps to increase weight in very few days.
7. Eating Coconut everyday helps to increase weight.
8. Boil Dry Dates (Chuhara) in Milk and drinking this regularly helps to increase weight.
9. Eating Peas (Mutter) in meals also helps to increase weight.
10. Eating Groundnut (Moong phali) regularly helps to increase weight.

11. Regular body massage helps to increase weight for underweight people.

12. Eating Black gram (Urad) in any form helps to increase weight.

13. Dip few Californian raisin (Monakka) in water and eat them along with water before going to bed or Milk boiled with few Californian raisins, mixed with Honey can be taken for few days helps to increase weight.

14. Dip 10 Almonds (Badam) overnight and peel the skin in the morning, add some Butter and Sugar and eat this everyday which helps to increase weight.

15. Drinking Carrot juice regularly helps to increase weight.

16. Eat lot of ghee, milk products, sweets etc which helps to increase weight.

17. Mix boiled Rice with plain Curd in the night and keep it. Eat this in the morning in empty stomach for few days to increase weight which is also good for Eyes and Migraine.

Chapter 34

Increase Breast Milk

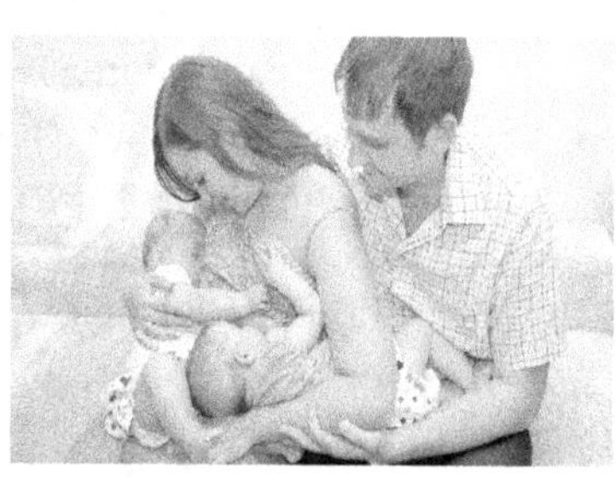

Breastfeeding is a pleasant experience both for the mother and the child. It is also very much needed for the developing a loving bond between mother and the child. The breast milk has all the nutrients essential for the child's growth. During the baby's first year it is very much needed to provide the child with the essentials ingredients to build up his/her immunity system. But most mothers suffer from the lack of milk production.

If you have reason to believe that your supply of breast milk has decreased, then you may be wondering how to increase breast milk. A dwindling of breast milk supply may be due to a multitude of things, such as too much stress, baby's increased demand due to a growth spurt, or not enough feedings. If this is making you feel down, do not worry. There are lots of remedies in getting you to increase your supply of breast milk, and fortunately, they're not that hard to follow.

Remedies to Increase Breast Milk
1. Dip few Fenugreek seeds (Menthi) in water for few hours, then boil it till the seeds are smooth and this can be taken with Milk after delivery helps to increase breast milk.
2. Use of Black gram (Urad) in any form like Dal, Idli, etc helps in increasing breast milk.

3. Drinking Carrot juice regularly helps to increase breast milk.
4. Eating raw Onion along with meals helps to increase breast milk.
5. Eating Roasted Cumin seeds (Jeera) with Sugar twice a day after delivery helps to increase breast milk.
6. Eating Grapes also helps to increase breast milk.
7. Taking boiled Drumstick (Muranka Bhaji) leaves during pregnancy helps to increase breast milk later on.
8. Massaging breasts with Castor oil (Erand) in the starting weeks of delivery also helps to increase breast milk.
9. Eating Musk melon (Kharbooja) also helps to increase breast milk.
10. Eating Peas (Mutter) in any form helps to increase breast milk.
11. Leaves of "Touch me not" (Lajavanti) plant grinded and applied on the breasts helps to increase breast milk.
12. Grind Shatavari (Asparagus racemosus) root, mix this paste with Milk and Sugar and filter. Drinking this Milk helps to increase breast milk.
13. Mukuna wanna or Water Amaranth (Gudrisag in Hindi or Honagonne in Kannada) leaves grinded and 4 spoons of this juice added with 2 spoons of Honey and taken everyday after delivery helps to increase breast milk.
14. Drinking Milk boiled with Cumin seeds (Jeera) and mixed with Honey, regularly during pregnancy helps to increase breast milk.

Chapter 35

Increase Memory Power

Brain power and memory plays a key role in day to day life of person. Healthy lifestyle with good diet and regular exercises helps to a great extend in improving memory power.

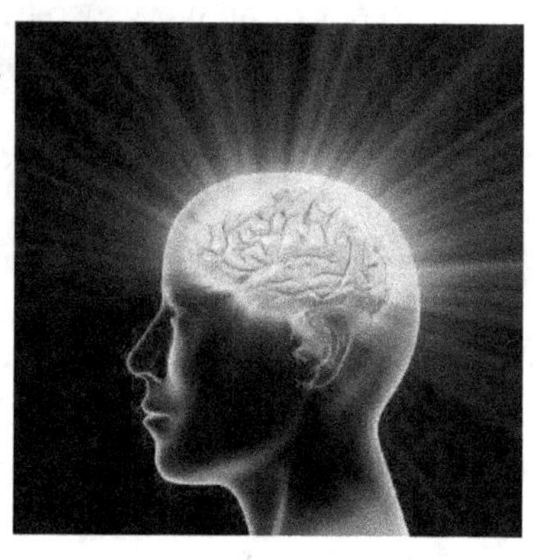

Patients with poor memory focus are advised to include a good amount of antioxidants, vitamins, omega 3 and whole grains in their diet. Improving oxygen consumption of cells, increasing the energy level of person and promoting blood circulation throughout the body are other health benefits of consuming herbal remedies for poor brain power and memory.

Remedies to Increase Memory Power

1. Brahmi (Gotu kola) is said to be very good for brain. Children can take a spoon of Brahmi juice and adults can chew 5-6 Brahmi leaves everyday to increase memory power. It is an antioxidant which reduces brain aging.
2. Eating 10 Almonds (Badam) in empty stomach everyday morning helps to increase memory power.
3. Eating Gooseberries (Amla) or its Morabba everyday morning helps to increase memory power.
4. Eating an Apple everyday, 15 minutes before meals helps to increase memory power.
5. Eating Walnuts (Akhroat) regularly helps to increase memory power.

6. Cinnamon (Dalchini) powder mixed with Honey can be taken everyday to increase memory power.

7. Drinking Ash gourd (Petha) juice everyday helps to increase memory power.

8. Drinking hot Milk mixed with Cardamom (Elaichi) powder and Honey, everyday helps to increase memory power.

9. Eating Coriander (Dhania) powder mixed with Honey before sleep helps to increase memory power.

10. Eating Raw Fenugreek (Menthi) leaves mixed with small pieces of Radish (Muli), Salt and Cumin (Jeera) powder also helps to increase memory power.

11. Eating Cashew nut (Kaju) everyday also helps to increase memory power.

12. Sesame seeds (Til) are rich in protein and said to be very helpful in increasing memory power. A Sweet ball (laddoo) can be prepared with Sesame seeds and Jaggery (Gur) and taken everyday.

13. Drinking Wheat grass juice is very good for health and helps to increase memory power.

14. Mango milkshake (Aam ras) and Honey taken regularly helps to increase memory power.

15. Eating Ginger piece with few Cumin seeds (Jeera) and Sugar candy (Mishri) helps to increase memory power.

16. Taking Black pepper powder with pure Butter helps to increase memory power.

17. Drinking Carrot juice everyday morning helps to increase memory power.

18. Ghee (prepared from cow milk) massaged on the head and 2-3 drops of pure Ghee put in the nostrils everyday also improves memory power.

19. Black berry (Jamun) is also very helpful in increasing memory power.

20. Urad dal (Split horse bean) can be taken with Ragi Rotis also helps in increasing memory power.

Chapter 36

Increase Immunity/ Resistance Power

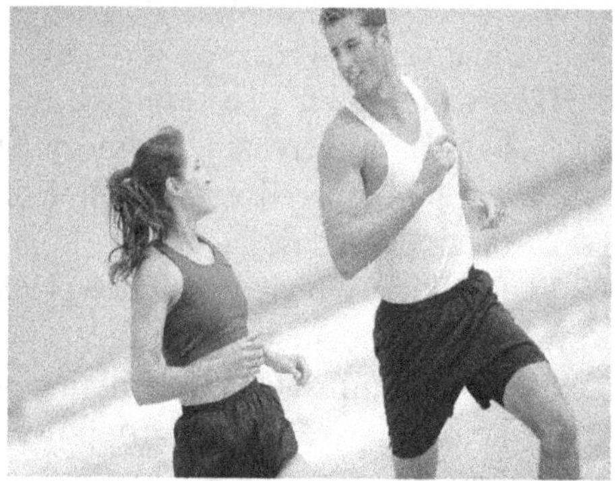

Ayurveda relates the body's immunity to Ojas— that is the essence of the seven tissues that make up the body. The ancient Indian therapeutic science strongly counsels that we take care of the Ojas or the vital energy for good health and wellbeing.

The seven tissues or dhatus are believed to make up the human body. These are Rasa [juice], Rakta [blood], Mansa [muscle], Medha [body fat], Asthi [bones], Majja [bone marrow] and Shukra [semen]. Ojas, the prime source of natural immunity, is the core extract of these seven body tissues and is highly vital to life and existence.

Ojas is the end product of complete digestion that creates radiant good health, stable emotions, and immunity. Ama, the digestive impurities caused by eating hard-to-digest foods or by unhealthy eating habits, creates the opposite effect--it compromises immunity and health.

Remedies to Increase Immunity/Resistance Power

1. Drinking Luke warm water mixed with a spoon of pure Honey and a spoon of Lemon juice everyday morning helps to increase resistance power.

2. Drinking Milk boiled with a pinch of Turmeric and Black pepper (Kali mirch) every night before going to bed prevents many diseases and also helps to increase resistance power.

3. Eating a Gooseberry (Amla) everyday helps to improve resistance power by providing necessary vitamins and iron.

4. Eating 5 Basil (Tulsi) leaves everyday helps to increase resistance power even for Cancer

5. Drinking Milk boiled with Harad (Haritaki) powder and mixed with a spoon of Honey everyday helps to increase resistance power.

6. Eating Papaya (Papita) everyday helps to increase resistance power.

7. Betel leaves (Pan) with small quantity of Lime (Chuna) and a piece of Areacanut (Supari) taken helps to increase resistance power.

Chapter 37

Indigestion

When we are not able to digest a particular food or when we overeat then we have indigestion problem with symptoms of nausea, stomach pain, Heaviness etc. Causes may be too much spicy, heavy foods, eating too fast, eating with anger and anxiety, allergic to some foods etc. Some 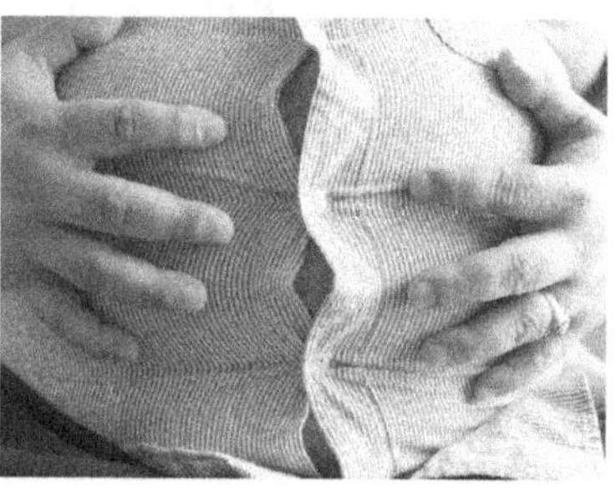 home remedies are given below which helps to overcome indigestion problem.

Remedies for Indigestion

1. A spoon of Carrom seeds (Ajwain) and Black salt taken with hot water reduces indigestion.
2. Drinking salted Buttermilk everyday helps to reduce indigestion.
3. Eating a piece of Ginger after every meals helps to prevent indigestion problem.
4. Lemon juice with Black salt taken with Luke warm water also helps to cure indigestion problem.
5. Using Garlic or Asafoetida (Hing) in meals also helps to reduce indigestion.
6. Eating a Banana after every meals helps to overcome indigestion problem.
7. Eating White grapes regularly helps to overcome indigestion problem.

8. Eating Papaya (Papita) everyday also helps to improve digestion and prevents indigestion problems.

9. Eating Radish with Salt and Black pepper (Kali mirch) along with meals also helps in curing indigestion problem.

10. Equal quantities of Cinnamon (Dalchini), Dry ginger (Saunth), Cardamom (Elaichi) powdered, eating a pinch of this powder helps in curing indigestion.

11. Eating Orange with Black salt after meals helps to get relief from indigestion problem.

12. When you are facing indigestion due to drinking plain milk, add a Long pepper (Pipple) or Ginger piece (Adrak) or few Cumin seeds (Jeera) while boiling milk.

13. Drinking Mint (Pudina) juice with Honey every morning helps to overcome indigestion problem.

14. Eating Drumstick (Muranka Bhaji) in any form helps to reduce indigestion problem.

15. Drinking a spoon of Honey helps to reduce indigestion.

16. Makoy leaves and fruits are very good for digestion. Eat them regularly to overcome indigestion problem.

17. Brinjal (Byangan) especially long one is good for curing indigestion problem.

18. Eating a Gooseberry (Amla) everyday helps to prevent indigestion problem.

19. Eating a piece of Jaggery (Gur) after meals helps to overcome indigestion problem.

20. Drinking a spoon of Basil (Tulsi) juice helps to overcome indigestion problem.

21. Boil Asafoetida (Hing) in water and drink it or applying Asafoetida paste on the naval helps in curing indigestion problem.

22. Boil Cloves (Laung) in water and drink it which also helps to prevent indigestion problem.

23. Sitting in Vajrasan for 5 minutes after every meal is very good for curing indigestion problem.

24. Applying few drops of Mustard (Sarson) oil inside the naval regularly helps in curing indigestion problem.
25. Eating Aniseed (Sauf) after every meals helps to cure indigestion problem.
26. Back berries (Jamun) are very good for digestion. Eat them regularly to overcome indigestion problem.
27. Eating Guava (Amrud) with Salt helps in curing indigestion problem.
28. Taking Roasted Cumin seeds (Jeera) with Honey helps in curing indigestion problem.
29. Eating Roasted Onion or raw Spring onion (Pyaj ka Phool) are helpful in curing indigestion problem.
30. Using Sweet Neem (Curry patta) regularly in cooking helps to overcome indigestion problem.
31. Eating a Cardamom (Elaichi) after meals also helps to overcome indigestion problem.
32. Eating Sugar cane (Ganna) after meals helps to digest the food and cures indigestion.
33. Eating Bitter gourd (Karela), White goose foot (Bathua) leaves in any form helps to overcome indigestion problem.
34. Eating Black pepper (Kali mirch) powder with Lemon juice and hot water helps to reduce indigestion problem.
35. Drinking a spoon of raw Potato juice helps to reduce indigestion problem.

Chapter 38

Injury/Cuts

Injury/Cuts are wounds that break through the skin, and sometimes reach the underlying tissue. Scratches are usually superficial wounds where the skin is scraped by a sharp object.

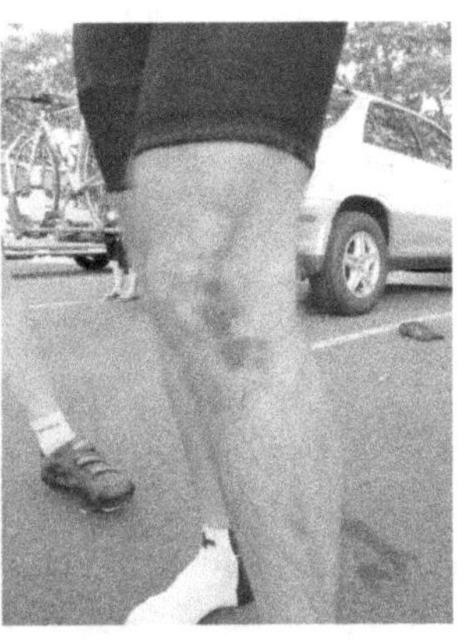

The skin is a barrier between the environment and the rest of the body. Usually it offers protection from the invasion of infective organisms. If the skin is broken by cutting or scratching, there is an increased possibility of infection, along with pain and blood loss. Most cuts and scratches are relatively minor and respond well to home remedies. Deep cuts may require medical help and repairing the skin with stitches to heal properly.

Remedies for Injury/Cuts

1. Any type of injury small or big, applying Neem oil is the best and wonderful remedy which protects the wound from infection and helps the wound to heal very fast.
2. Mango leaf burnt and its ash mixed with Honey, this paste applied on the injury stops bleeding immediately.
3. Ice piece (Baraf) rubbed lightly on the injured area stops bleeding immediately.
4. Durva (Dub, grass used to worship Lord Ganesha) juice applied on the injury helps to stop bleeding immediately.
5. Applying Gooseberry (Amla) juice on the injury stops bleeding immediately.

6. Applying juice, oozed from a cut on raw Banana, on the injury helps to heal the injury faster.

7. Applying grinded Neem leaves paste on the injured area helps to heal the injury faster and prevents infection.

8. Applying Honey on the injured area helps to heal injury faster and remove its scars.

9. Applying juice, oozed from a cut on raw Papaya (Papita), on the injury helps to heal the injury faster.

10. Thick skin of raw Papaya tied on the injury helps to heal the injury faster.

11. Applying raw Potato paste on the internal blood clot (Blue colour) due to an injury is helpful to reduce the pain.

12. Drinking hot Milk mixed with a spoon of Turmeric powder is very good remedy for any type of internal injury.

13. Tamarind (Imli) pulp heated and applied on the swelling caused by an internal injury helps to heal the injury faster and reduces the pain.

14. Applying the paste of Carrom seeds (Ajwain) grinded with Lemon juice on the swelling caused by an internal injury helps to cure the injury faster and reduces pain

15. Sandalwood paste applied on the swelling caused by an internal injury helps to cure the injury faster and reduces pain.

16. A piece of cloth dipped in a mixture of Onion juice and Turmeric powder, applied over the swelling caused by an internal injury, helps to heal the injury faster.

17. The swelling caused due to an internal injury can be heated, with the help of hot Salt tied in a cloth, which reduces the swelling and pain.

18. The swelling caused due to an internal injury can be heated, with the help of heated Drum stick (Muranka bhaji) leaves tied in a cloth ,which reduces the swelling and pain.

19. Applying Turmeric paste on the swollen or sprained area, caused due to internal injury, helps to reduce pain and swelling.

Chapter 39

Insomnia

Insomnia is a condition in which person finds difficulty in getting sleep or disturbed sleep. Causes of insomnia can be mental tension, lack of physical activity, over eating, health problems, irregular routine etc.

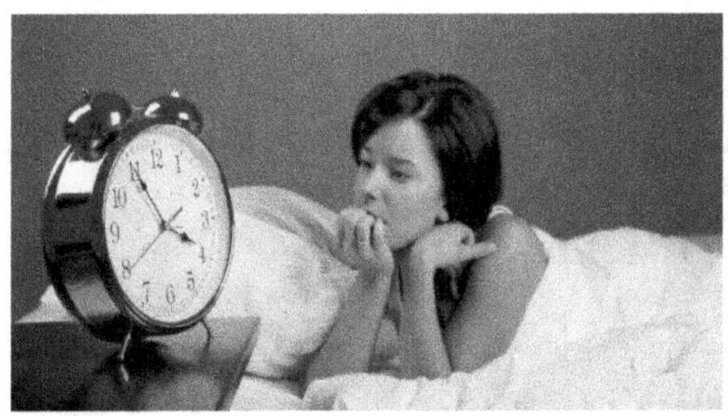

Prevention

1. Establish a regular bed and rising time.
2. Drink at least 10 glasses of water each day.
3. Take healthy diet; avoid alcohol, tobacco, stimulants like coffee, tea, especially before sleep.
4. Listening to some light music, reading a book of interest, creative thinking, and chanting gods name helps in getting sleep.
5. Go for hot water bath or a body massage before sleep.
6. Sufficient physical activity or exercise during day time can help in getting good sleep during night.
7. Avoid watching TV for long hours.
8. Resist napping during day.
9. Do not skip meals during day and avoid eating late.

10. Ensure that the bed is comfortable and the environment relaxing.

Remedies for Insomnia

1. Massaging foot sole with Mustard (Sarson) oil before going to bed helps to overcome Insomnia.
2. Poppy seeds (Khus Khus) dipped in water for an hour, grinded to form a paste. Boil this paste with Milk and Sugar. Drinking this is very effective to overcome Insomnia.
3. Eating Mango and drinking Milk or drinking Mango milkshake (Aam ras) regularly in the night helps to overcome Insomnia.
4. Eating a raw Onion or roasted Onion in the night also helps to get rid of Insomnia problem.
5. Nut Meg (Joy phal) powder mixed with water taken in the night helps to overcome Insomnia.
6. Consuming lot of Curd or eating Curd with Sugar or sweet Lassi induces sleep and cures Insomnia.
7. Drinking hot Milk with a spoon of Ghee and Sugar in the night helps to get sleep and cures Insomnia.
8. Drinking a glass of Carrot juice everyday helps to cure Insomnia.
9. Drinking a spoon of Lemon juice mixed with a spoon of Honey in the night induces sleep and cures Insomnia.
10. Coriander (Dhania) leaves grinded with water and mixed with Sugar and eating this paste helps to get sleep and cures Insomnia.
11. Aniseeds (Sauf) boiled in water for 10 minutes, add Milk and Sugar. Drinking this before going to bed helps to get rid of Insomnia problem.
12. Cucumber (Kheera) piece rubbed on the foot sole makes a cooling effect on the body and helps to get sleep curing Insomnia.

13. Putting Castor oil (Erand) on the head or body massaged with Castor oil regularly helps in curing Insomnia.

14. Sprouted Horse gram (Kulthi) taken regularly helps to get sleep and cures Insomnia.

15. Consuming Dry fruits and Oat regularly helps to cure Insomnia.

16. Indian gooseberry (Amla) helps to improve the body's immune system by providing necessary vitamins and iron. Eating this everyday helps in curing Insomnia.

Chapter 40

Itching

Itching on a body can be because of many reasons. Sometimes it can be side effect of some medicines, some diseases or it can be due to insect bites, allergies, dry skin, blood disorders, impure blood, Thyroid problems, pregnancy, diabetes, use of cosmetics. Here are some 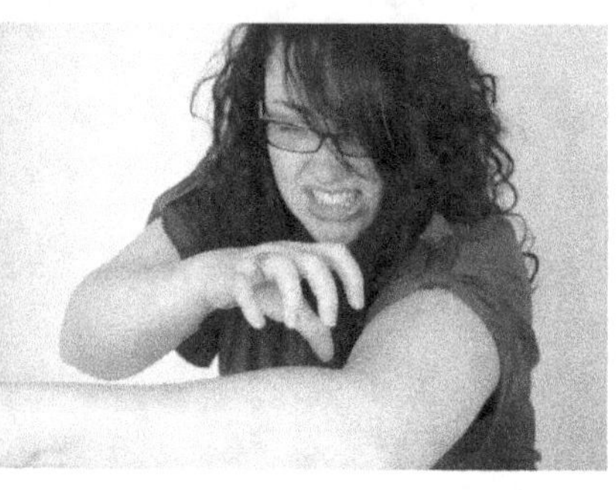 home remedies in general. Salt and sugar should be avoided during Itching problem.

Remedies for Itching

1. Drink one tablespoon of hot pure Ghee in one go, empty stomach in the morning, for few days to cure Itching problem. Ghee should be hot enough but bearable.
2. Boil Neem leaves in sufficient water for 10-15 minutes. Taking bath with this water helps in curing many skin diseases including Itching.
3. Durva (Dub, A grass used to worship Lord Ganesha) juice mixed with Turmeric powder applied on the affected area cures Itching.
4. Bottle gourd (Ghea) juice applied on the affected area cures Itching.
5. Boil some Coriander (Dhania) seeds in water and add Sugar and filter. Drinking this decoction helps to reduce Pitt and Itching.

6. Drinking Mint (Pudina) juice and applying Mint juice on the body also cures Itching.

7. Applying the paste of grinded Tender Guava leaves and Curd, on the body 2 hours before taking bath helps to cure Itching.

8. Eating raw Cabbage (Patta gobi) everyday helps to cure Itching.

9. Boil some Cumin seeds (Jeera) in water and taking bath with this water helps to cure Itching.

10. Applying Milk on the body before taking bath also helps to get rid of Itching problems.

11. Banana pulp meshed with Lemon juice applied on the affected area helps to cure Itching.

12. Drinking few drops of Neem juice or applying Neem oil on the affected area helps to cure Itching.

13. Basil (Tulsi) juice mixed with Lemon juice applied on the body helps to stop Itching.

14. Mix two spoons of Coconut oil with one spoon of Tomato juice, this oil can be applied on the body before taking bath (with warm water) reduces Itching.

15. Taking 10 whole Black peppers (Kali mirch) powder with a spoon of Ghee, twice a day for few days cures Itching.

16. Harad (Haritaki) powder boiled in water to form a paste, this paste applied on the body with the help of a cloth cures Itching.

17. Garlic cloves boiled in any type of oil (used for body message), this oil applied on the affected area reduces Itching.

18. Pigeon pea (Arhar dal) grinded and mixed with Curd, applied on the body reduces Itching.

19. Coconut oil mixed with small quantity of Lemon juice, applied on the affected area helps to reduce Itching.

20. Eating boiled White goose foot (Bathua) leaves for few days or washing affected area with its juice, reduces Itching.

21. Mix around 10 grams of Camphor (Kapoor) mixed with 100 grams of Coconut oil. This oil applied on the body reduces Itching.

22. Green gram (Moong) paste applied on the affected area cures Itching.

23. Grinded Carrom (Ajwain) leaves applied on the body, half an hour before taking bath helps to cure Itching.

24. Drink milk mixed with grinded Carrom (Ajwain) leaves and Sugar, which helps to cure Itching.

Chapter 41

Low Blood Pressure

When the pressure of the blood in the arteries goes abnormally lower than the normal then it is said to be low blood pressure or hypotension. During this, blood flow to the brain and other organs will not be sufficient which leads to dizziness, giddiness, even fainting. It may be due to infection, weakness, too much medication, too much medicine for hypertension, pregnancy etc. It can be cured with natural home made remedies. During Low blood pressure Salt intake should be increased.

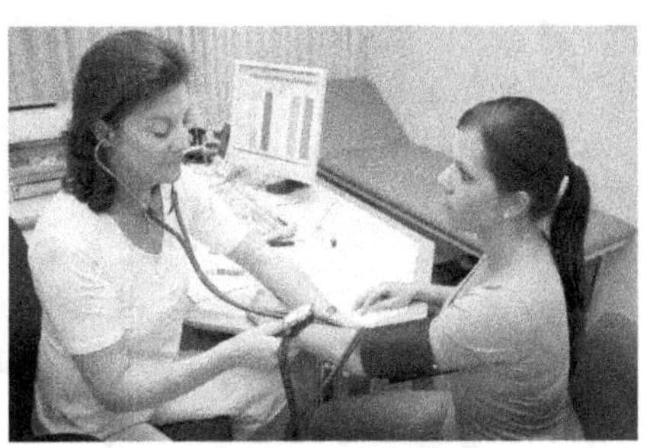

Remedies for Low Blood Pressure

1. Drinking Beetroot juice every day helps to control Low blood pressure.
2. Chewing 4-5 Basil leaves (Tulsi) with a spoon of Honey in the morning helps to control Low blood pressure.
3. Dip 5-10 Raisins (Kishmish) overnight in water. Eat Raisins with water in the morning which helps to control Low blood pressure.
4. Dip 10 Almonds (Badam) in water overnight, remove the skin in the morning. Eat these almonds empty stomach which helps to control Low blood pressure.
5. Mint (Pudina) juice helps in controlling blood pressure. Drinking Mint juice regularly helps to cure Low blood pressure problem.

Chapter 42

Malaria

Malaria is an acute infectious disease caused by parasitic infection of red blood cells and transmitted through mosquitoes. The symptoms are chills, high fever, headache, vomiting, tiredness, nausea, diarrhoea, sweating. Malaria fever starts with chills and ends with sweat. Malaria fever comes every alternate day or after every few days. How often the fever returns varies.

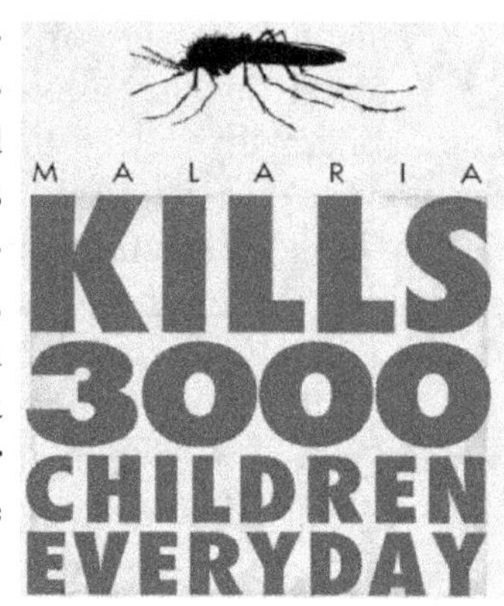

Remedies for Malaria

1. Boil Cinnamon (Dalchini) and Black pepper (Kali mirch) in water and filter. Drink this hot decoction mixed with Honey, which reduces fever and chills during Malaria.
2. Boil Orange skin in water for 20 minutes and filter. Drink this hot decoction, which is helpful during Malaria.
3. Basil (Tulsi) leaves rubbed on the body reduces chills during Malaria.
4. Drink one spoon of Lemon juice with one spoon of Onion juice thrice a day, which reduces fever during Malaria.
5. When fever repeats every fourth day during Malaria, drinking Lemon juice in water with sugar daily, reduces fever.
6. A Lemon piece filled with Salt and Black pepper can be heated and sucked slowly, twice a day, which is helpful during Malaria.

7. When fever repeats every fourth day during Malaria, drinking Buttermilk (Chach) helps in fast recovery.

8. Eating Banana, Guava (Amrud), Apple during Malaria helps in fast recovery.

9. Equal quantities of Coriander (Dhania) powder and Dry ginger powder (Saunth) can be mixed, eating a spoon of this mixture thrice a day with water helps to reduce fever during Malaria.

10. Take Long pepper (Pipple) powder mixed with Honey, which reduces fever during Malaria.

11. Boil Neem leaves and Black pepper (Kali mirch) in water and filter. Drinking this decoction helps to cure Malaria.

12. Boil Basil (Tulsi) leaves and Black pepper powder in water and filter. Drinking this decoction helps to cure Malaria.

13. Boil one spoon of Black pepper powder, three Garlic cloves in one cup of water and filter. Drinking this decoction (after cooling) with a spoon of honey, thrice a day helps to cure Malaria.

Chapter 43

Menstrual Stomach Ache

Stomach ache during menstrual period is so common in girls. Some female get pains even a week before menstruation begins and some female face severe pain just before the menstruation. It is advisable to eat light diet with more fruits and vegetables and avoid spicy chilled foods, specially during that period. Here are some home remedies to get relief from stomach ache due to menstrual period.

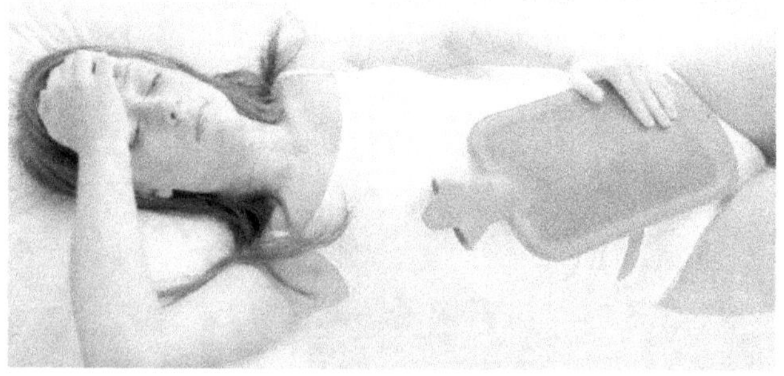

Remedies for Menstrual Stomach Ache

1. Eating a pinch of Asafoetida (Hing) kept inside a Banana fruit pulp or Asafoetida with Jaggery and drinking hot water helps to reduce stomach ache during menstruation.
2. Eating a spoon of Fenugreek seeds (Menthi) with a cup of Buttermilk (Chach) helps to reduce stomach ache during menstruation.
3. Eating Black Sesame seeds (Til) powder with hot Milk during menstruation helps to get relief from stomach ache.

4. Putting a wet cloth on the naval area cools the stomach helps to reduce stomach ache during menstruation.

5. Dry Ginger (Saunth) and Jaggery (Gur) boiled in water, filtered and drinking this decoction helps to reduce stomach ache during menstruation.

6. Drinking Half spoon of Neem leaf juice mixed with one fourth spoon of Ginger juice helps to reduce stomach ache during menstruation.

7. Mustard seeds powdered and boiled in water. A cloth dipped in this hot solution can be put on the stomach which helps to reduce stomach ache during menstruation.

8. Eating Carrom seeds (Ajwain) and jaggery (Gur) with pure Ghee helps to reduce stomach ache during menstruation.

9. Aniseeds (Saunf) boiled in water, filtered and drinking this decoction with a spoon of Honey helps in reducing stomach ache during menstruation.

10. Guava fruit (Amrud) pulp without seeds mixed in Milk with Honey, taken reduces stomach ache during menstruation.

11. Eating Radish and Radish leaves helps in controlling stomach ache during menstruation.

12. Black Cotton leaves grinded and mixed with Milk, drinking this milk helps in reducing stomach ache during menstruation.

Chapter 44

Migraine

Migraine is a severe headache, usually affecting one side of head, with nausea, eye pain, giddiness, vomiting, visual disturbances etc. Migraine can be because of many reasons like mental tensions, allergies, tiredness, anger, Eye strain, indigestion, sudden change of weather etc.

Remedies for Migraine

1. Mix plain Rice with Curd in the night and keep it overnight. Eat this rice in the morning in empty stomach for some days to cure Migraine.
2. Massage head with Castor oil (Erand) and put a wet cloth on the fore head, both helps to get relief from Migraine pain.
3. Eating a spoon of Honey with half spoon of Salt or just eating Honey or putting Honey in nostrils all helps to cure Migraine pain.
4. Eating Jaggery (Gur) mixed with Pure Ghee, (Ghee prepared from cow milk) in the empty stomach for 5 days to helps to cure Migraine.
5. Eating Goose berries (Amla) with Salt gives relief from Migraine.
6. Eating Apple pieces with Salt for 3 weeks helps to get permanent relief from Migraine.
7. Apply diluted Asafoetida (Hing) paste on the forehead and

try to inhale its smell, to get relief from Migraine. Don't rub it as it can cause skin irritation.

8. Mustard (Sarson) oil drops put in the nostrils (If you are having left side pain put in the right nostril and vice versa) for few months helps to get permanent relief from Migraine.

9. A few drops of Ghee prepared from cow milk put in the nostrils (If you are having left side pain put in the right nostril and vice versa) for few months helps to get permanent relief from Migraine.

10. Drinking a spoon of Basil (Tulsi) juice mixed with Honey helps to get relief from Migraine.

11. Eating some sweet or Sugar or jaggery during Migraine reduces pain in some people instantly.

12. Chewing some Black pepper (Kali mirch) with pure Ghee (Ghee prepared from cow milk) helps to get relief from Migraine.

13. Dry Ginger (Saunth) mixed in water can be smelled and applied on the forehead (avoid rubbing) reduces Migraine pain.

14. Putting Drum stick leaves (Muranka Bhaji) juice in the nostrils (If you are having left side pain put in the Right nostril & vice versa) gives relief from Migraine.

15. Smelling Onion juice or chewing raw Onions helps to get relief from Migraine pain.

16. 5 drops of Drum stick leaf juice and Ginger juice equally mixed and filtered can be put in the ear (If you are having left side pain put in the Right ear and vice versa) to get relief from Migraine pain.

17. Putting few drops of Almond (Badam) oil in the nostrils for some days helps to get permanent relief from Migraine.

Chapter 45

Mouth ulcer

Mouth ulcer is a painful bubble inside the mouth on lips, tongue, gums etc. These can be small, large or in clusters. These create burning and pain. Causes of mouth ulcer are due to nutritional deficiencies, infection, allergic to some medicines, excess stomach heat etc.

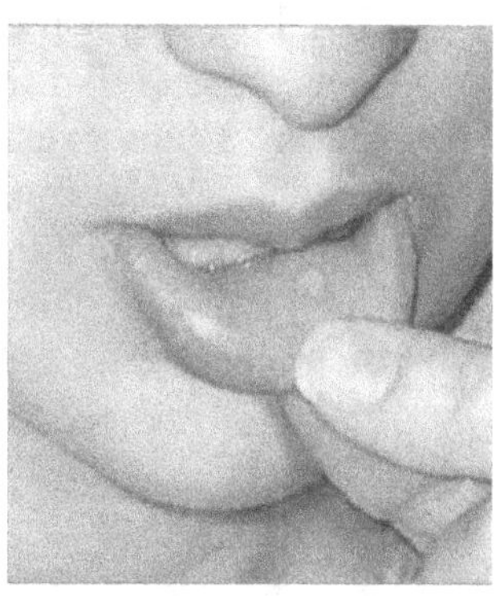

Remedies for Mouth ulcer

1. Applying Honey or pure Ghee or Glycerin on the bubbles helps to cure Mouth ulcer faster.
2. Eating Banana mixed with Curd in the morning gives instant relief from Mouth ulcer.
3. Slowly chewing Vaali leaf (Basale soppu in Kannada) gives a quick relief from Mouth ulcer.
4. Eating a raw Tomato or washing mouth with Tomato juice helps to cure Mouth ulcer.
5. Durva (Dub, a grass used to worship Lord Ganesha) boiled in water, filtered and this decoction used as a mouth wash cures mouth ulcers.
6. Washing mouth with Warm Bitter gourd (Karela) juice mixed with a pinch of Alum powder (Phitkari) or only Bitter gourd juice, gives relief from Mouth ulcer.
7. Warm water mixed with Salt and Lemon juice used as a mouth wash helps to get relief from Mouth ulcer.
8. Tender Guava (Amrud) leaves boiled in water with Salt and

filtered. This decoction used as a mouth wash cures Mouth ulcer.

9. Gooseberry (Amla) leaves boiled in water and filtered. Washing mouth with this decoction helps to cure Mouth ulcer faster.

10. Harad (Haritaki) powder mixed with Honey applied on the bubbles helps to cure Mouth ulcer.

11. Chewing Poppy seeds (Khus Khus) with dry Coconut or dry Coconut with Sugar candy (Mishri) helps to get relief from Mouth ulcer.

12. Camphor (Kapoor) with pure Ghee can be applied on the bubbles and washed later. This can be done 2-3 times a day to get relief from Mouth ulcer.

13. Chewing Henna (Mehandi) leaves, or Henna leaves boiled in water and filtered, and use of this decoction as a mouth wash, helps in curing Mouth ulcer.

14. Boil Turmeric powder in water and this warm decoction used as a mouth wash helps in curing Mouth ulcer.

15. Pomegranate (Anar) skin boiled in water, filtered and this decoction used for washing mouth gives a great relief from Mouth ulcer.

16. Chewing Mint (Pudina) leaves gives relief from Mouth ulcer.

17. Chewing Makoy leaves gives quick relief from Mouth ulcer.

18. Drinking Goat milk or fresh milk just after milking cow (without boiling) helps to get relief from Mouth ulcer.

19. Eating boiled Ragi everyday prevents Mouth ulcer as it keeps the stomach cool.

20. Eating Aniseeds (Sauf) after meals prevents Mouth ulcer.

21. Boil Coriander seeds (Dhania) in water and filter. Washing mouth with this decoction or just applying Coriander leaves paste on the bubbles gives relief from Mouth ulcer.

22. Drinking Gooseberry juice with Cumin powder (Jeera) and Buttermilk (Chach) or drinking Gooseberry juice with Honey helps in curing Mouth ulcer.

Chapter 46

Nose Bleeding

Epistaxis or Nose bleeding is a common problem which can be treated with simple home remedies. The causes are nose picking with some sharp object, allergy, cracks in the nostril due to dryness, cold, excessive heat in the body etc.

Remedies for Nose Bleeding

1. Putting a piece of Ice (Baraf) on the head or putting a wet cloth on the head is a good remedy to stop nose bleeding or Epistaxis.
2. Putting a drop of Lemon juice in both the nostrils, helps to stop nose bleeding or Epistaxis immediately.
3. Lie down putting your head backside with some pillows and then put 2-3 drops of pure Ghee in the nostrils and try to inhale slowly which helps to stop nose bleeding or Epistaxis.
4. Putting Onion juice drops in the nostrils, helps to stop nose bleeding or Epistaxis.
5. Putting Neem juice drops in the nostrils, helps to stop nose bleeding or Epistaxis.
6. Smelling Cow dung helps to stop nose bleeding or Epistaxis.
7. Drinking Durva (Dub, a grass used to worship Lord Ganesha) juice mixed with Sugar, stops nose bleeding or Epistaxis.
8. Black Cotton leaves grinded and squeezed to extract juice, this juice applied on the centre of the head, stops nose bleeding or Epistaxis.

9. Putting Sweet grape juice in the nostrils helps to stop nose bleeding or Epistaxis.
10. Use of Gooseberry (Amla) is a good remedy to cure nose bleeding or Epistaxis. Drinking Gooseberries juice with water or applying Gooseberries paste on the centre of the head or Gooseberries juice put in the nostrils, all are helpful to stop nose bleeding or Epistaxis.
11. Putting Pomegranate (Anar) juice in the nostrils, stops nose bleeding or Epistaxis.
12. Putting Basil (Tulsi) juice in the nostrils cures nose bleeding or Epistaxis.
13. Eating a piece of Coconut everyday in the empty stomach, helps to overcome nose bleeding or Epistaxis.
14. Black gram (Urad dal) grinded with water and this paste applied on the forehead helps to stop nose bleeding or Epistaxis.
15. Drinking Ash Gourd (Petha) juice everyday keeps the body cool and stops nose bleeding or Epistaxis.
16. Dip 2 Figs (Anjeer) in water overnight. Eating them with water in the morning, helps to overcome nose bleeding or Epistaxis problem.
17. Drinking milk with a spoon of pure Ghee helps to stop nose bleeding or Epistaxis.

Chapter 47

Obesity

Obesity is nothing but deposition of extra fats which later may leads to many health problem like heart attack, high blood pressure, diabetes etc. Over weight makes extra pressure on the heart, kidney and other vital organs and their functioning, ultimately affecting the life span. Causes of Obesity are improper metabolism, overeating, lack of physical activity, improper digestive system, hereditary problems, eating fried and junk foods, sleeping in excess, menstrual problems, thyroid problem etc.

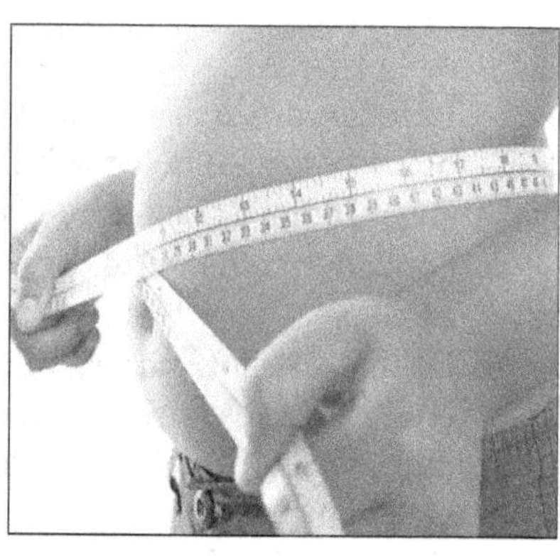

Remedies for Obesity

1. Avoid fried items, sweets, chocolates, ice creams, ghee, oil etc. Eat healthy foods like fruits, vegetables, sprouts etc to avoid Obesity.

2. Doing regular exercise like long walk in the morning and evening, yoga and other physical exercise will reduce extra accumulated fat thereby reducing Obesity.

3. Drinking a glass of hot water with a spoon of Lemon juice and a spoon of Honey in the morning is a good remedy for fighting Obesity.

4. Bitter gourd juice (Karela) taken in the morning can do wonders in case of Obesity by reducing excess fat considerably.

5. Eating raw Tomatoes and Onion with a pinch of Salt everyday helps to remove extra fat and reduce Obesity.

6. Eating ten raw Sweet Neem (Curry patta) leaves everyday, reduces fat and Obesity.

7. Eating Radish (Muli) daily, helps to reduces fat and Obesity.

8. Substitute Rice and wheat with Ragi, which helps to reduces fat and Obesity.

9. Chewing Garlic everyday in the empty stomach with a spoon of Honey, helps to reduces fat and Obesity.

10. Massaging the body at least once in a week, helps to reduces fat and Obesity.

11. Fasting or taking only fruit diet one day in a week also helps to reduce Obesity.

12. Drinking Ash gourd (Petha) juice regularly, helps to reduces fat and Obesity.

13. Eating Triphala powder (Triphala is composed of Harad (Haritaki), Indian gooseberries (Amla) and Behada (Bibhitaki)) every night before going to bed, helps to reduces fat and Obesity.

14. Taking Steam bath once in a week, helps to reduces fat and Obesity.

15. Drinking a spoon of Cow urine everyday morning, helps to reduces fat and Obesity.

16. Eating Drumstick (Muranka Bhaji) or Drumstick leaves regularly in meals, helps to reduces fat and Obesity.

17. Banana grinded in Milk and mixed with a spoon of Banana flower Juice. Taking this for 80 days will definitely reduce weight and cures Obesity.

18. Eating Cucumber (Kheera) daily helps to reduces weight and Obesity.

19. Dinking Buttermilk (Chach) everyday helps to reduce weight and Obesity.

20. Eating raw Cabbage (Patta gobi) everyday helps to reduce weight considerably and Obesity.

21. Drinking Spinach (Palak) juice with Lemon juice regularly helps to reduce weight and Obesity.

Chapter 48

Piles

Piles are an inflammation and enlargement of veins in the rectum area. Piles may be internal or external.. Piles arise from the exerted force for passing stool which causes pressure on the veins. It is a piece of flesh hanging out of rectum which will be very painful. Although Piles is not a major problem and this can be handled 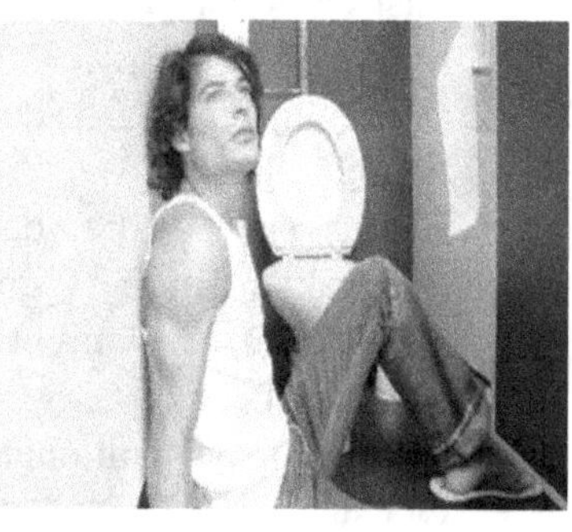 with simple home remedies, severe cases requires even surgery. Better to cure in the initial stage. The main cause of Piles are chronic constipation. Other than this, the causes includes eating lot of chilies, drinking less water, prolonged sitting, obesity, mental tensions, too much heat in the body etc. Symptoms are severe pain and burning or bleeding in flesh piece hanging outside rectum during passing stools. Even otherwise also it can cause irritation, itching, pain, burning in the rectum area, difficulty in sitting etc. Avoid chilly as much as possible, Treat constipation, drink lots of water.

Piles are categorized in two types.
1. Bleeding Piles
2. Non bleeding Piles

Remedies in General for Both Bleeding and Non Bleeding Piles
1. Radish (Muli) is very helpful in curing Piles. Regularly eating raw Radish or drinking Radish juice with a spoon of ghee helps to reduce Piles problem.

2. Drinking a spoon of Ginger juice mixed with 2 spoon of Mint (Pudina) juice and 4 spoons of Honey 3 times a day, helps in curing Piles.

3. Equal quantities of Haritaki (Harad), Long pepper (Pipple), Sugar candy (Mishri) powdered, and half spoon of this powder taken with Butter, both in morning and evening, for some days helps to cure Piles.

4. Taking 10 milliliter of Onion juice mixed with a spoon of Sugar for 15 days, helps in curing Piles.

5. Drinking Aloe Vera (Gwar Patha) juice for few days helps in curing Piles.

6. Elephant foot corn (Jimi kand) pieces powdered and 5 grams of this powder taken with Ghee, Honey and Jaggery (Gur) or taken with Buttermilk for few days, also cures Piles.

7. Eating boiled Raw Banana without skin regularly, helps to cure Piles.

8. Eating Onion pieces with Jaggery (Gur) or eating spring onions (Pyaj ka Phool) are very good for Piles.

9. Drinking Butter milk with a half spoon of Turmeric powder helps in curing Piles.

10. Drinking Sweet Neem (Curry patta) juice with Honey or Sweet neem juice with Buttermilk helps to cure Piles.

11. Eating raw Bitter gourd (Karela) or drinking Bitter gourd juice helps to cure Piles.

12. Regularly eating Dates (Khajur) helps to cure Piles.

13. Eating a spoon of Neem seed powder with Honey everyday, helps to cure Piles.

14. Eating a spoon of Roasted Sesame seeds (Til) with Jaggery (Gur) for few days, helps to cure Piles.

15. Eating Papaya (Papita) everyday helps to cure Piles.

16. Using Banana stem regularly in cooking is beneficial in Piles.

17. Eating Black berries (Jamun) or drinking Black berries juice with Honey helps to cure Piles.

18. Eating a Banana with a Cardamom (Elaichi) everyday helps to cure Piles.

19. Eating 4-5 Neem flowers with Sugar candy (Mishri) in empty stomach for few days helps to cure Piles.
20. Eating cabbage (Patta gobi) is also very beneficial in curing Piles.
21 Eating Colcasia (Arbi) is also helpful in curing Piles.

Remedies for Bleeding Piles

1. Put Lemon juice in hot Milk. Drinking this immediately, thrice a day, helps to cure bleeding Piles.
2. Equal quantities of Onion, Black pepper (Kali mirch), Basil (Tulsi) leaves grinded together and half spoon of this taken, both in morning and evening for few days, will definitely cure bleeding Piles.
3. Taking dry Gooseberries (Amla) powder with hot Milk every morning helps to cure bleeding Piles.
4. Radish (Muli) is very helpful in curing Piles. Regularly eating raw Radish or drinking Radish juice with a spoon of ghee helps to reduce Piles problem.
5. 20 Gram of Coriander (Dhania) powder boiled in water for 15 minutes and filtered. This decoction taken with Milk and Sugar for few days cures bleeding Piles.
6. Eating boiled Raw Papaya (Papita) or eating ripe Papaya regularly, helps to cure bleeding Piles.
7. Bottle guard (Ghea) skin can be dried and powdered. Taking a spoon of this powder with water twice a day helps to cure bleeding Piles.
8. Eating Onion pieces with Jaggery (Gur) or eating spring onions (Pyaj ka Phool) are very good for bleeding Piles.
9. Eating grinded Coriander (Dhania) leaves with Sugar candy (Mishri), twice a day, helps to stop bleeding in Piles.
10. Eating tender Tamarind (Imli) leaves with Black pepper and raw Mango helps to stop bleeding in Piles.
11. Drinking Bitter gourd (Karela) juice with Sugar regularly helps to cure bleeding Piles.
12. Eating Lentil (Masoor dal) everyday and drinking sour Buttermilk helps to cure bleeding Piles.

13. Eating a spoon of Roasted Sesame seeds (Til) with Jaggery (Gur) everyday helps in curing bleeding Piles.

14. Eating Boiled Fenu greek seeds (Menthi) in Milk or Fenu greek sprouts are helpful in curing bleeding Piles.

15. Boil Cumin seeds (Jeera), Aniseed (Sauf), Coriander seeds (Dhania) in water for few minutes. Add pure Ghee and drink this, both in morning and night, which helps to cure bleeding Piles.

16. Dip some Figs (Anjeer) in water overnight and eat them empty stomach in the morning, which helps to cure bleeding Piles.

Remedies for Non Bleeding Piles

1. Applying Castor oil (Erand) or Mustard (Sarson) oil on the hanging flesh gives quick relief in Piles.

2. Applying "Tiger balm " or " Sensur ointment " on the hanging flesh helps to get relive from pain in Piles. Initially for few minutes it will burn but afterwards a cooling effect will be observed.

3. Eating Ridge gourd (Touri), Amaranth (Cholayi), White goose foot (Bathua leaves), Beet root, Elephant foot corn (Jimi kand), Cabbage (Patta gobi) all are very helpful in curing Piles.

4. Leaves of Bottle guard (Ghea) grinded and this paste applied on the hanging flesh gives relief from pain and cure Piles.

5. Radish (Muli) is very helpful in controlling Piles. Regularly eating raw Radish or drinking Radish juice with a spoon of ghee helps to reduce Piles problem.

6. Yellow portion of Aloe Vera (Gwar Patha) plant mixed with equal amount of Castor oil (Erand) kept under sun for some time, will harden like wax .This wax applied on the hanging flesh will be very helpful in curing Piles.

7. Sitting inside a big bucket containing Luke warm water everyday or regular boating helps to cure Piles.

8. Drumstick leaves (Muranka Bhaji) and Radish leaves grinded together, this paste applied on the hanging flesh helps to cure Piles.

9. Rice flour and Turmeric powder mixed in water to make a paste and this paste applied on the hanging flesh helps to cure Piles.

10. Tea leaves grinded in water, this paste applied when hot on the hanging flesh helps to relive from pain and cures Piles.

11. Eating Onion pieces with Jaggery (Gur) or eating Spring onions (Pyaj ka Phool) are very good for Piles.

12. Drinking Carrot juice or Spinach (Palak) juice helps to cure Piles.

13. Eating Guava (Amrud) everyday helps to cure Piles.

14. Wheat grass juice taken everyday helps to cure Piles.

15. Eating half spoon of Dry ginger (Saunth) powder with Jaggery (Gur) twice a day helps to cure Piles.

16. Taking Harad (Haritaki) with hot water is also beneficial in curing Piles.

17. Drinking Butter milk (Chach) with Rock salt (Saindha namak) everyday will be helpful in curing Piles.

18. Eating Sugar candy (Mishri) with Cumin seeds (Jeera) or eating Aniseeds (Sauf) everyday gives relief from Piles.

19. Eating 4-5 Neem flowers with Sugar candy (Mishri) in empty stomach for few days helps to cure Piles.

Pneumonia

Pneumonia is a lung infection caused by bacteria, virus, parasite. Symptoms are severe cold, cough, unusual rapid breathing, fever, vomiting, stomach pain, wheezing sound, loss of appetite etc. Pneumonia occurs more in children than elders. It is advisable to consult a qualified doctor immediately after getting the Pneumonia symptoms.

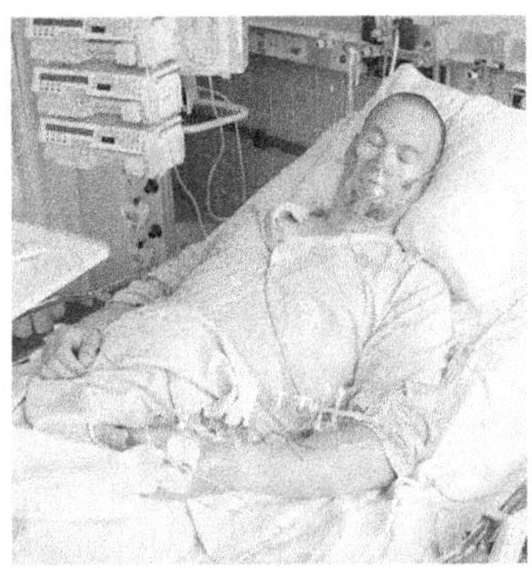

Remedies for Pneumonia

1. Garlic is said to be very good for Pneumonia. 5 drops of garlic juice in 2 spoons of hot water should be taken during Pneumonia.
2. Applying external heat to chest, by hot water bag or heated salt tied in a cloth makes the breathing easier during Pneumonia.
3. Taking a pinch of Asafoetida (Hing) in warm water gives relief during Pneumonia.
4. Boil few Basil leaves with Black pepper (Kali mirch) in water and filter. Drinking this decoction helps in Pneumonia.
5. Drinking Honey mixed with warm water during Pneumonia gives strength and helps for easy digestion.
6. In case of excessive wheezing sound during Pneumonia, Boil five whole Black peppers with five Californian raisins (Monakka) in water for some time and filter. A spoon of this decoction taken thrice a day helps to reduce Balgum (Phlegm).

Chapter 50

Poisonous Bites

There are insects like mosquitoes, which suck our blood and leave a tiny wound on our skin, on biting. On the other hand there are bees and wasps whose stings contain venom. Mostly these bites and stings last for a day or two but people differ in their reactions.

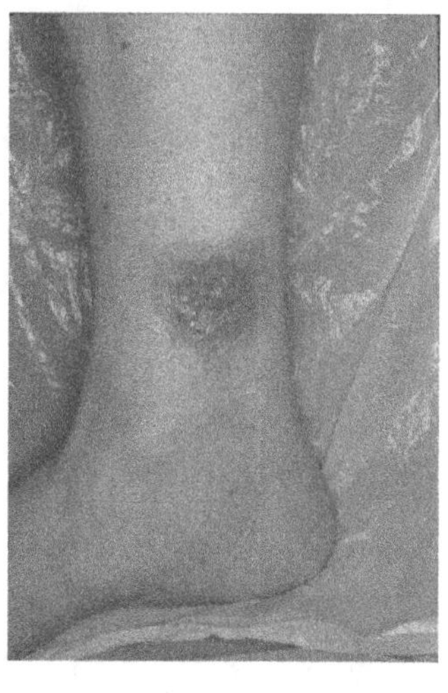

Some people get allergies after these insect bite or sting which leads to redness, swelling or pain and itching. While some people are prone to a very serious reaction to a venom which shows swelling of the airways. Rocky Mountain spotted fever and Lyme disease are caused by the mosquitoes but this is restricted to some parts of the world.

You can take some precautions to avoid these bites and stings. You should cover your skin in the insect bite prone area. Try to screen the windows and doors. Insects can be kept away by applying five drops of citronella mixed in a cup full of water on the uncovered skin areas.

Remedies for Poisonous Bites

1. Applying Lemon juice mixed with Salt on the affected area helps in reducing the effect of poisonous bite.
2. Applying Onion juice mixed with Honey on the affected area helps in reducing the effect of poisonous bite.

3. Applying Garlic paste on the affected area helps in removing the poisonous effect of a poisonous bite.

4. Pomegranate (Anar) leaves grinded and its juice applied on the affected area helps in reducing the effect of poisonous bite.

5. Applying Asafoetida (Hing) paste on the affected area helps in reducing the effect of poisonous bite.

6. Applying Neem leaf juice on the affected area helps in reducing the effect of poisonous bite.

7. Applying Mint juice on the affected area helps in reducing the effect of poisonous bite.

8. Ash gourd (Petha) stalk grinded with Sandal wood and this paste applied on the affected area helps in reducing the effect of poisonous bite.

Chapter 51

Prickly Heat

Prickly heat is nothing but the small itchy rashes or boils caused by sweat entrapped under the skin.

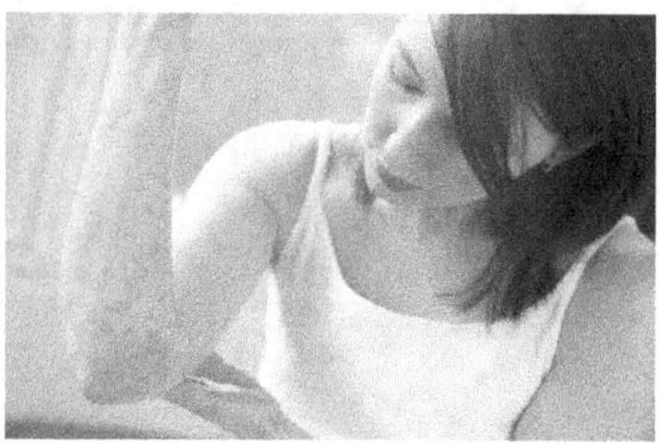

Remedies for Prickly heat

1. Washing the affected parts with discarded water during washing Rice, gives relief from prickly heat.
2. Brinjal (Byangan) pieces dipped in water for some hours. This water used to wash the affected area gives relief from prickly heat.
3. Taking bath only with cold water also helps to get relief from prickly heat.
4. Applying Henna paste (Mehandi) gives a quick relief from prickly heat.
5. Massaging the body with Gingery (Til) oil also helps to get relief from prickly heat problem.
6. Fenugreek seeds (Menthi) dipped in water and later grinded with Coconut to form a paste. Applying this paste on the whole body and head half an hour before taking bath, gives relief from prickly heat.

7. Applying Harad (Haritaki) powder mixed in water on the body before taking bath helps to get relief from prickly heat.

8. In stead of using soap go for Soap nut (Shikakai) or Gram flour (Besan) which helps in controlling prickly heat.

9. Applying Goose berry (Amla) paste on the affected parts, gives relief from prickly heat.

10. Applying Bitter gourd (Karela) juice mixed with small quantity of eating Soda on the affected parts, gives relief from prickly heat.

Chapter 52

Pyorrhoea

Pyorrhoea is a disease of gums. It affects the membrane surrounding the roots of the teeth and leads to loosening of the teeth, pus formation, and shrinkage of the gum.

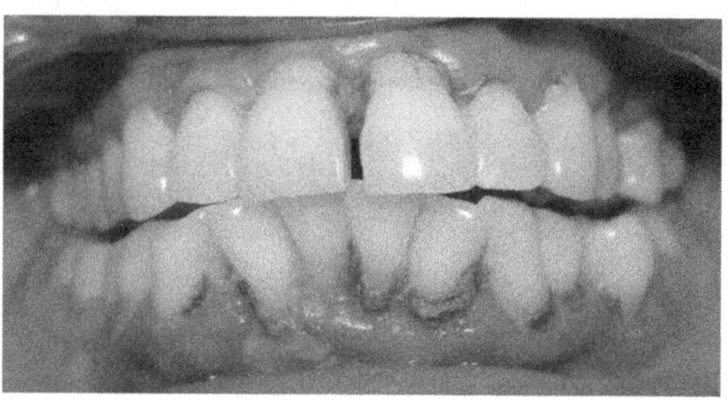

Remedies for Pyorrhoea

1. Rubbing Rock salt (Saindha namak) mixed with Mustard (Sarson) oil on the teeth regularly helps to cure Pyorrhoea.
2. Drink lot of Orange juice and Carrot juice regularly to cure Pyorrhoea.
3. Tender Mango leaves boiled in water and filtered and this decoction used as a mouth wash regularly cures Pyorrhoea.
4. Regularly Rubbing Camphor (Kapoor) mixed with Castor oil (Erand) on the gums twice a day helps to cure Pyorrhoea.
5. Chewing raw Spinach (Palak) and drinking Spinach juice regularly, helps to overcome Pyorrhoea.
6. Cardamom (Elaichi) boiled in water and filtered, and this decoction regularly used as a mouth wash cures Pyorrhoea.
7. Orange skin dried and powdered and this powder regularly rubbed on the teeth helps to cure Pyorrhoea.

8. Regularly applying mixture of Lemon juice and Honey on the teeth cures Pyorrhoea.

9. Regularly applying Sandal wood paste on the teeth helps to cure Pyorrhoea.

10. Chewing Lettuce leaves everyday after meals helps in preventing Pyorrhoea.

11. Chewing unripe Guava (Amrud) is good for teeth and gums. Chewing tender guava leaves helps to cure bleeding gums. Guava root bark boiled in water and filtered, and this decoction used as a mouth wash cures swollen gums.

Chapter 53

Scorpion Bites

A scorpion is a small creature, about 6-10 cm long. It has a segmented body, with two poisonous glands in its tail. It holds its victim with its claws and pushes forward the tail and injects the poison into the body.

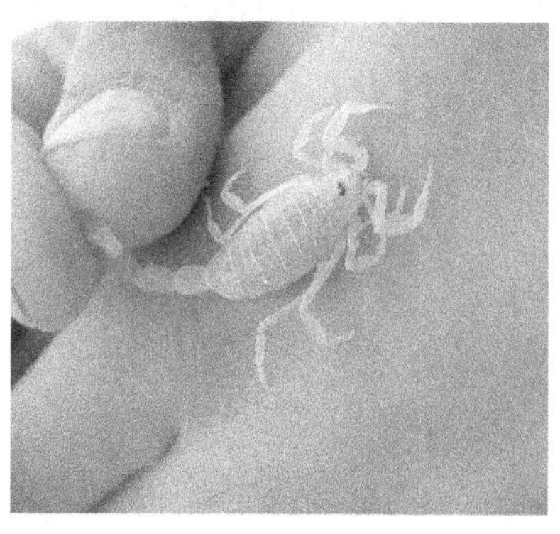

The scorpion is nocturnal in nature, i.e. it moves around during the night. During the day it remains hidden in various dark places, like in shoes, in clothes/bedding, on the ground, behind the furniture, they are also found in various cracks in the walls, and under rocks, in vegetation/ gardens, etc.

They usually move about during the warm season and, therefore, scorpion-stings are likely to occur more in summer, during the night.

Usually they do not jump and sting a person. They bite when someone comes into contact with them, or disturbs them. Children, being ignorant, while catching scorpions, may get bitten.

Remedies for Scorpion Bites

1. Applying Radish (Muli) paste mixed with Salt on the affected area and eating Radish helps in reducing the effect of scorpion bite.
2. Applying Onion juice on the affected area helps in reducing the effect of scorpion bite.

3. Applying Basil (Tulsi) leaves grinded with Salt on the affected area helps to reduce the pain during scorpion bite.

4. Applying Garlic paste on the affected area and drinking a spoon of Garlic juice with Honey helps in reducing pain and burning during scorpion bite.

5. Lemon seeds grinded and applied on the affected area gives relief from the burning and the pain during scorpion bite.

6. Applying Mint (Pudina) paste on the affected area and drinking Mint juice during scorpion bite is beneficial.

7. Applying Bottle guard (Ghea) paste on the affected area and drinking Bottle guard juice helps in removing poison of scorpion bite. .

8. Carrom (Ajwain) seeds grinded and applied on the affected area reduces the burning and the pain during scorpion bite.

9. Applying Apple paste on the affected area and eating Apple during scorpion bite is very helpful.

10. Pomegranate (Anar) leaves grinded and this paste applied on the affected area of scorpion bite is very helpful.

11. Alum (Phitkari) dissolved in water and applied on the affected area of scorpion bite is very helpful.

12. Tamarind (Imli) seeds crushed into pieces and dipped in water for sometime. These swollen seeds lightly pressed still it sticks, to the affected area of scorpion bite. These seeds will fall down itself after sometime after removing poison from the wound.

13. Grind dried Ash gourds (Petha) stalks with water to make a paste. Apply this paste on the affected area and heating the area with hot water bottle, helps in removing poison as well as reducing pain due to scorpion bite.

Snake Bites

There are many types of snakes and their poison intensity differs. It is very necessary to treat the snake bite immediately even though some snakes are less poisonous. When the snake bites, it is better to observe which type of snake it is as medicines are also different for different snake bites.

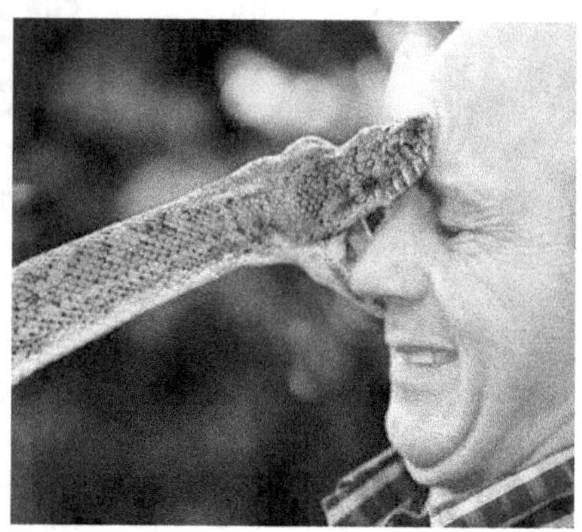

Remedies for Snake Bites

1. One Castor leaf (Erand) and 10 whole Black peppers (Kali mirch) grinded together and given immediately, causes vomiting and removes poison of the snake bite from the body. Repeat it number of times.
2. Drinking Banana stem juice is very effective remedy to remove poison from the body due to snake bite.
3. Chewing Neem leaves with Salt and Black pepper (Kali mirch) is helpful in removing poison of snake bite. If it tastes sweet, it is an indication of presence of poison in the body, and if it tastes bitter it indicates that the absence of poison in the body.
4. Taking grinded Basil (Tulsi) leaves with water helps during snake bite.

Chapter 55

Stammering

Stammering is nothing but inability to pronounce certain letter or words and disruption of flow of speech by repetition and prolongation of sounds. Other than children adults also suffer from Stammering. The causes are not clear till today but it can be due to heredity, tension and other factors.

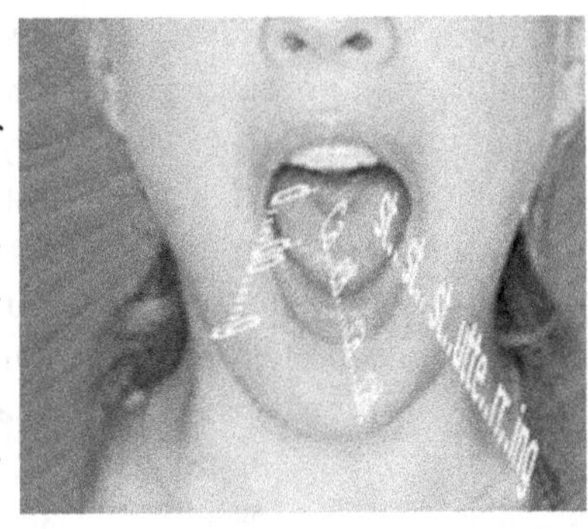

Remedies for Stammering

1. Eating a fresh Gooseberry (Amla) daily is helpful in curing stammering. A spoon of dry Gooseberry powder with a spoon of pure Ghee taken in the morning is also helpful in curing Stammering.

2. Dip 12 Almonds (Badam) overnight and peel them in the morning. Grind them and eat with 30 grams of pure butter. Continue this for few months to overcome Stammering.

3. Grind 10 Almonds and 10 whole Black peppers (Kali mirch) with a piece of Sugar candy (Mishri) and take it for some days to overcome Stammering.

4. Eating dry Dates (Chuhara) before going to bed but avoid drinking water for at least 2 hours, also helps to clear the voice and cures Stammering.

Chapter 56

Tooth Ache

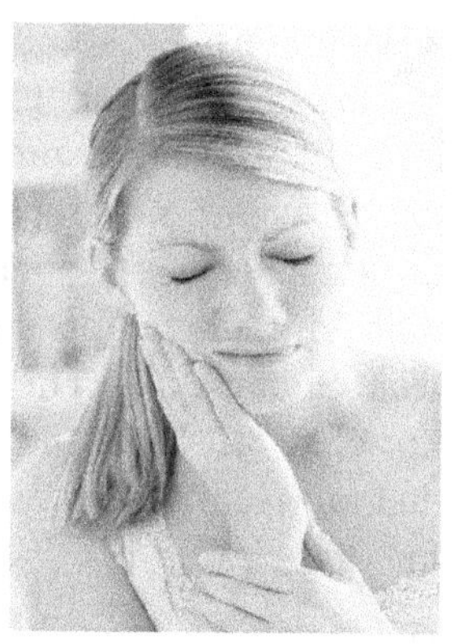

Tooth ache pain. You can't live with it, but you can definitely live without it. Depending on the root cause of your tooth ache, you may find it hurts just to move your head or even to breathe when air rushes past a sensitive area. Most of the time, it doesn't just hurt. It's pure agony. When you're in need of toothache pain relief and seeing the dentist isn't an option because of time or money, what can you do?

When looking for relief from tooth ache pain, your home, and more importantly your kitchen and bathroom, can be your best friend. There are a large number of natural home remedies for tooth ache, but virtually all are only temporary solutions. Sometimes that's all you need.

One of the advantages to home remedies is they are natural, inexpensive, don't have side effects, and won't cause you to become addicted like prescription pain killers can.

Remedies for Tooth Ache

1. Cotton dipped in Raw Papaya (Papita) juice applied on the affected tooth, reduces tooth ache immediately.
2. Keeping a piece of Onion on the affected tooth reduces tooth ache.
3. Washing mouth with Hot water mixed with Salt gives relief from tooth ache.

4. Boil few tender Mango leaves in water and washing mouth with this water, reduces tooth ache.

5. Put a piece of crushed Clove or a cotton piece dipped in Clove oil on the affected tooth, gives relief from tooth ache.

6. Keeping a piece of Tobacco on the affected tooth reduces pain in case of severe tooth ache.

7. Boil Neem leaves in water and washing mouth with this water, reduces tooth ache.

8. Put a piece of Camphor (Kapoor) or camphor piece dipped in Gooseberry (Amla) juice on the affected tooth, reduces tooth ache.

9. Boil some fresh Guava (Amrud) leaves in water and washing mouth with this water, or simply chewing fresh Guava leaves, helps to reduce tooth ache.

10. Roast a piece of Turmeric and powder it. Applying this on the affected tooth or applying Turmeric powder or a small piece of Turmeric kept on the affected tooth gives relief from tooth ache.

11. A roasted Garlic with Salt can be put on the affected tooth helps in reducing tooth ache.

12. Putting a piece of Asafoetida (Hing) on the affected tooth, helps to reduce tooth ache.

13. Basil (Tulsi) leaves grinded with Black pepper (Kali mirch) applied on the affected tooth gives relief from tooth ache.

14. Boil few Carrom (Ajwain) seeds in water and washing mouth with this warm water and keeping the warm water on the affected teeth for some time helps in reducing tooth ache.

15. Putting ground Mint leaves (Pudina) with Salt on the affected tooth, reduces tooth ache.

16. Boil Cardamoms (Elaichi) in water and washing mouth with this water helps in reducing tooth ache.

17. If pure home made Butter is available, make a small ball and wrap it with cotton. Applying this ball on the affected tooth for sometime cures tooth ache.

Chapter 57

Typhoid

Typhoid is an acute and infectious illness transmitted by contaminated water or food. Its symptoms are High fever, weakness, stomach ache, lack of appetite, body rashes, diarrhea, chills and body ache.

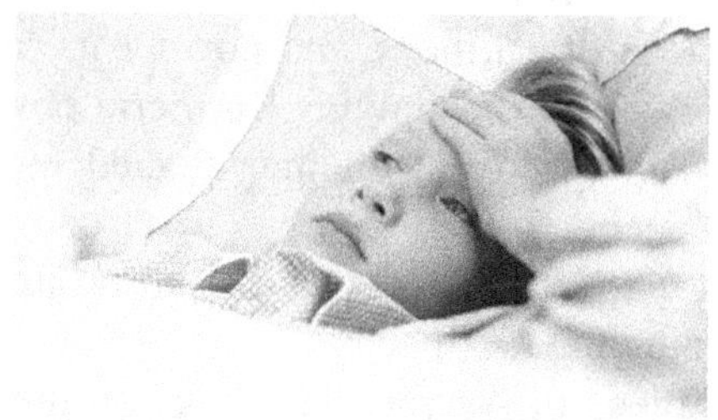

Remedies for Typhoid

1. Drinking Sweet lime (Mosambi) juice is beneficial during Typhoid.
2. Eating Banana pulp mixed with Buttermilk reduces fever during Typhoid.
3. Eating Californian raisin (Monakka) helps to kill Typhoid causing bacteria's.
4. Boil five Cloves (Laung) in water for 10 minutes filter. Drinking this decoction after cooling twice a day helps to get relief from Typhoid.
5. Eating Orange and milk, thrice is also beneficial during Typhoid.
6. Drinking hot water mixed with a spoon of Honey is helpful during Typhoid.
7. Drinking Apple juice is also advisable during Typhoid.

Chapter 58

Vomiting

Vomiting can be due to many reasons like gastric, poisonous intake, motion sickness, pregnancy, allergic to some drugs, very bad smell, very dirty or scary scene etc.

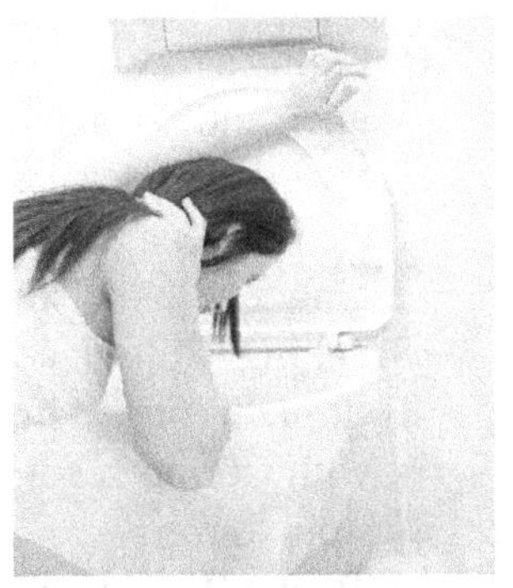

Remedies for Vomiting

1. Drinking Lemon water or smelling a Lemon while traveling is the best solution to stop vomiting due to motion sickness.
2. Eating Orange with Salt preferably Black salt helps to stop vomiting caused by motion sickness.
3. Ripe Banana is helpful during blood stains in the vomit.
4. A pinch of Powdered Clove (Laung) with Honey taken helps to stop vomiting during pregnancy.
5. Eating Gooseberry (Amla) Morabba helps to stop vomiting during pregnancy.
6. Roasted Bengal gram (Chana) powdered and taken with water helps to reduce vomiting during pregnancy.
7. Drinking Water melon (Tarbooj) juice mixed with Sugar candy (Mishri) powder helps to stop vomiting caused by Pitt.
8. Drinking a spoon of Tamarind juice (Imli) helps to stop vomiting caused by Pitt.
9. Drinking Sugar cane juice (Ganna) juice with Honey helps to stop vomiting caused by Pitt.
10. Boil ground Coriander (Dhania) seeds or leaves grinded in water and filter. Sipping the decoction slowly helps to stop vomiting.

11. Drinking a spoon of Basil (Tulsi) juice with Honey helps to stop vomiting.

12. Boil Neem leaves in water and filter. Drinking this decoction helps to stop vomiting.

13. Eating Harad (Terminalia chebula, Haritaki) powder mixed with Honey helps to stop vomiting.

14. Drinking Mint (Pudina) juice mixed with Lemon juice helps to stop vomiting.

15. Putting some wet cloth on the stomach over the navel area cools the stomach and helps to stop vomiting due to Pitt.

16. Eating a raw Onion with Honey or drinking a spoon of Onion juice and Ginger juice, helps to stop vomiting.

17. Sprinkle Black pepper (Kali mirch) powder and Rock salt (Saindha namak) on a piece of Ginger. Slowly sucking the ginger helps to stop vomiting.

18. Taking Cumin seeds (Jeera) powder, Cardamom powder (Elaichi) mixed in a spoon of Honey, or drinking milk boiled with Cumin seeds powder and Cardamom powder, helps to stop vomiting.

19. Taking Powdered Cinnamon (Dalchini) mixed with Honey, or drinking milk boiled with Cinnamon, helps to stop vomiting.

20. Sucking a piece of Ice (Baraf) helps to stop vomiting.

21. In half glass of water put half spoon of Lemons juice, pinch of Cumin (Jeera) powder and a pinch of Cinnamon (Dalchini) powder. Drinking this thrice a day helps to stop vomiting.

22. Grind Black pepper (Kali mirch) with Onion and tie this in a clean thin cloth and hang it .The juice which drops from this cloth can be taken to stop vomiting.

23. Smelling roasted Clove (Laung) helps to stop vomiting sensation.

24. Boil two Cloves with a pinch of Cinnamon (Dalchini) in water and filter, drinking this decoction helps to stop vomiting.

Chapter 59

Warts

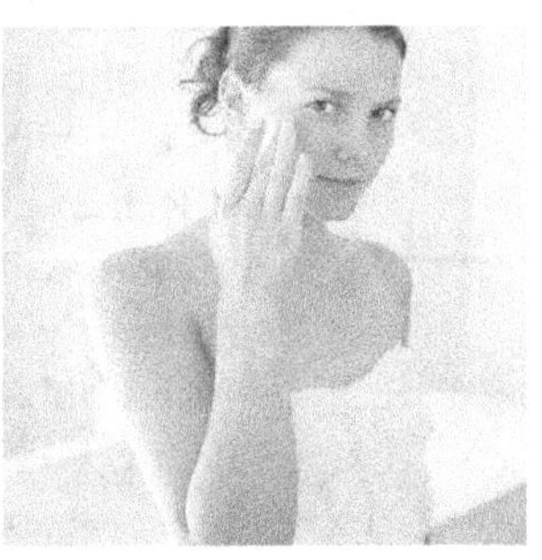

Warts are nothing but the extra elevations on the skin. Warts will appear more frequently on the fingers, elbows, knees, face, and scalp. Warts appearing on the soles of the feet are called plantar Warts. They are very painful and the person will not be able to walk properly. The main cause of Warts is virus infection of skin. All Warts are not painful but due to cosmetic reason people wants to get rid of them.

Remedies for Warts

1. Apply Castor oil (Erand) over the affected parts or Warts every night. The treatment should be continued for several months to get rid of Warts.

2. Cashew nut oil is useful in removing Warts. As it is a strong irritant to the skin, it should be applied externally over the affected areas.

3. Onions are irritating to the skin and stimulate the circulation of the blood. Warts sometimes disappear when rubbed with cut onions for few days.

4. Raw potatoes are useful for treating Warts. They should be cut and rubbed on the affected area several times daily, for at least two weeks.

5. Milky juice of a fresh Fig (Anjeer) applied on the Warts for two weeks helps to get rid of them.

6. Raw Papaya (Papita) juice or Pineapple juice applied on the Warts helps to get rid of them.

7. Applying Lemon juice on the Warts also helps to get rid of them. Covering the Wart with cotton dipped in Lemon juice continuously for some days, helps in smoothening and getting rid of Warts.

8. Mix baking soda with Castor oil and rub it on the Wart and cover it with a bandage. Repeat this every day. In a week or two, the Wart will swell and turn red. Keep repeating the application of the mixture till the Wart fall off.

9. Applying Sour tasted Apple juice on Warts for some days helps to get rid of Warts from the root itself.

10. Take a thin slice of fresh Garlic, large enough to cover the wart. Place it directly on wart and hold it with a plastic bandage. Remove bandage and garlic next day after bathing. A little blister will appear. Allow blister to be subside and dry away. Wart will fall in two weeks.

11. Eating raw Cabbage (Patta gobi) regularly for some days helps to get rid of Warts.

12. Applying Coriander paste (Dhania) on the Warts helps to get rid of them.

13. Rubbing a fresh Aloe Vera (Gwar Patha) leaf on the Warts for few days, helps to get rid from them.

Chapter 60

Worms

The Worms are present in the intestine, sometimes they come out with stool. Sometimes stools get stuck in the intestine which produces Worms. These may cause bloating, anemia, asthma, diarrhea, digestive disorders, fatigue, low immune system, nervousness, skin rash. Parasites Worms can invade your bodies through contaminated food and water intake, through a 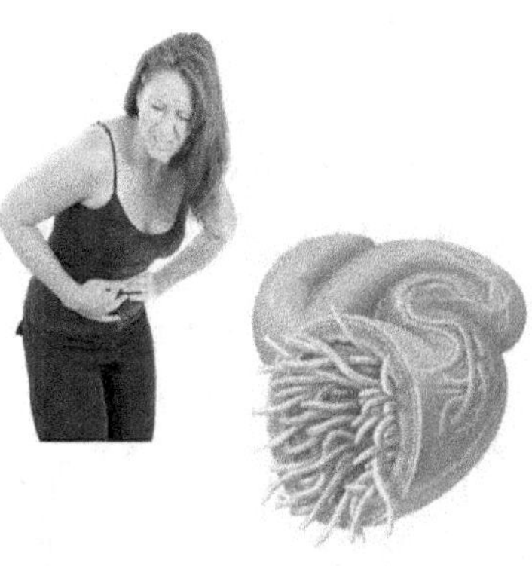 transmitting agent (like a mosquito), sexual conduct or through the nose and broken skin. Once established, they will start consuming the food and grow and slowly cause more problems to the body.

Remedies for Worms

1. Eating a pinch of roasted Asafoetida (Hing) mixed with a spoon of Lemon juice in the morning for 6 days, helps to get rid of Worms.
2. 10 seeds of ripe Papaya (Papita) grinded with 1/4th cup of water, taken for 7 days, helps to get rid of Worms.
3. Drinking salted Buttermilk in the morning is helpful in killing Worms.
4. Drinking Bitter gourd (Karela) juice or Bitter gourd juice with equal amount of Coconut milk for few days helps to get rid of Worms.
5. Drinking a spoon of Basil (Tulsi) juice for few days, helps in killing Worms.

6. Drinking Water mixed with few drops of Neem oil for few days, helps to kill Worms.

7. Boil a spoon of Coriander (Dhania) powder and Black pepper (Kali mirch) powder in water and filter. Drinking this decoction for few days, helps to get rid of Worms.

8. Drinking one spoon of Honey mixed with two spoons of Curd for few days, helps to kill Worms.

9. Drinking Pomegranate juice everyday also helps to kill Worms.

10. Drinking Coconut water and eating raw Coconut, both are useful in getting rid of Worms.

11. Drinking half cup of Mint juice (Pudina) for 7 days helps to kill Worms.

12. Sprinkle a pinch of Black pepper and Salt on red Tomatoes. Eating this tomato in the morning helps to kills Worms.

13. A spoon of Carrom (Ajwain) powder mixed with Jaggery (Gur), taken empty stomach for 3 days, helps in killing Worms.

14. Drinking a spoon of Onion juice once in 2 hours for few days helps to kill Worms.

15. Powder few Lemon seeds and mix it with 1/4 th cup of water. Drinking this for 7 days kills Worms.

16. Eating Apple in the night before going to bed and avoid drinking water the whole night. Repeating this for few days, helps to kill Worms.

17. Taking 2 grams of Mango seed powder with water for some days, helps to get to rid of Worms.

18. Drinking 2 spoons of Indian Gooseberry (Amla) juice for 5 days helps to get rid of Worms.

19. Drinking Carrot juice empty stomach for few days helps to get rid of Worms.

20. Drinking hot water, half an hour after every meal for 10 days, helps to kill Worms.

21. Eating half spoon of Salt before meals for 10 days, doesn't allow Worms to multiply, and also kills Worms.

22. Eating Lentil (Masoor dal) regularly for few days, doesn't allow Worms to multiply, and also kills Worms.

23. Taking 4 grams of Carrom (Ajwain) powder with a glass of Buttermilk for 7 days or taking 7 drops of Carrom oil helps in killing Worms.

24. Eating roasted Corn (Bhutta) once in a while doesn't allow Worms to develop.

25. Eating a pinch of Asafoetida (Hing) mixed with a spoon of fresh Neem juice before going to bed for 3 days, helps in killing Worms.

26. Eating few Ash gourd (Petha) seeds with Sugar for few days, helps to kill Worms.

27. Half spoon of Garlic juice mixed with a spoon of Honey taken for few days, helps to kill Worms.

28. Eating raw Papita (Papaya) with Sugar for few days destroys Worms.

29. One gram of Black pepper (Kali mirch) powder with Buttermilk taken for 7 days helps to get rid of Worms.

30. Eating a Wall nut (Akhroat) with Milk for few days, helps to kill Worms especially in children.

31. Eating Jaggery (Gur) before taking any allopathic medicine for killing Worms is very beneficial, as Worms sticking in the intestine wall will come out to eat Jaggery and get killed.

32. Eating Harad (Haritaki) is also a very good remedy for killing Worms.

Chapter 61

Wounds

Everyone comes across some or the other kind of wound every now and then. While the major ones are given due care and attention, and you rush to the nearest nursing home as soon as possible. The problem, however, arises many times with smaller ones.

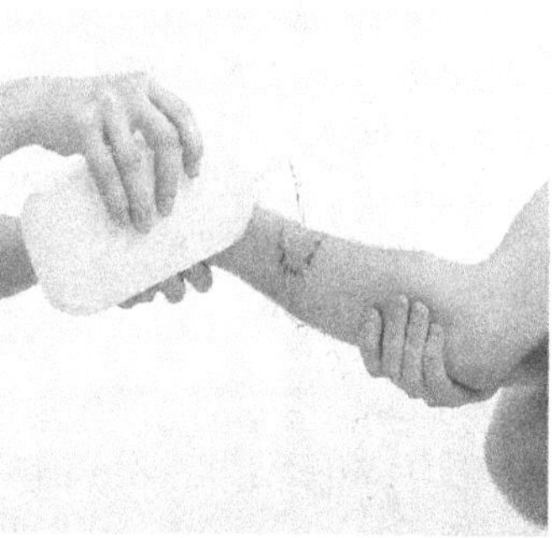

These wounds or abrasions are often caused when we are busy doing our house jobs, repairing the vehicle or cutting vegetables in the kitchen. Well, most of the times, you would ignore them or apply some cream or lotion on to the wound. You may also tend to use some readymade bandage to it and get going the other moment.

Many times, you are lucky enough and do not suffer from any serious consequences but this may not be the case all the time. The smaller looking wounds may put you in big trouble. Who knows you develop tetanus or any other kind of infection in that minor wound. Therefore you have to be cautious on this.

Remedies for Wounds

1. Applying Neem oil on any type of wounds cures the wound very fast.

2. Sesame seeds (Til) and Neem leaves roasted with Castor oil (Erand) and grinded with Turmeric and little Camphor, can be used as an home made ointment. Daily use of this ointment cures wound faster.

3. Eating oranges, garlic, grapes, carrots helps to heal the wounds faster.
4. Applying Honey on the wounds helps to heal the wound faster and also removes its scar.
5. Boiled Carrot pulp (after cooling) applied on the wounds, help to heal the wound faster.
6. Grinded Basil leaves (Tulsi) applied on the wounds heals the wound faster. Water boiled with Basil leaves can be used to wash wounds which helps to kill germs and prevent infection.
7. Applying Turmeric paste on the wounds and drinking Turmeric with milk helps to heal the wound faster and helps to kill germs and prevent infection.
8. Potato boiled in water and this water used to wash the internal wounds reduces swelling and pain.
9. Washing wounds with own Urine, helps to heals the wound faster and helps to kill germs and prevent infection.
10. Applying Sandal wood paste on the wounds helps to heal the wound faster.
11. Applying juice, oozed from a cut on raw Banana, on the wounds helps to heal the injury faster.
12. Applying juice, oozed from a cut on raw Papaya (Papita), on the wounds helps to heal the injury faster.
13. Garlic juice and Turmeric mixed with Gingery (Til) oil applied on the swelling helps to reduce swelling and heals wounds faster.
14. Tamarind (Imli) pulp heated and applied on the swollen area (internal injury), helps to cure the wounds faster and reduces pain.
15. Applying the paste of Carrom seeds (Ajwain) grinded with Lemon juice on the swelling caused by a wound helps to cure the wound faster and reduces pain.
16. The swelling caused due to a wound can be heated, with the help of hot Drum stick (Muranka bhaji) leaves tied in a cloth. This will reduce the swelling and pain.

17. Tie grinded Mint (Pudina) in a cloth and apply the cloth over the wounds, it helps to heal the wound faster and helps to kill germs and prevent infection.
18. Applying raw Potato paste on the internal blood clot (Neel, Blue colour), due to an internal injury, is helpful in reducing the pain.
19. Boil Camphor (Kapoor) in Coconut oil and apply this oil over the swollen area. Wash the swollen area with hot water next day. This helps to reduce swelling caused by an internal injury.

Chapter 62

Wrinkles

Wrinkles are the visible creases on the skin which is undesirable specially on the face. Usually wrinkles are connected with skin aging but premature wrinkles can be due to less water intake, continuous exposure to sunlight, skin problems, poor nutrition, stress, consuming alcohol, exposure to cigarette smoke, lack of sleep etc.

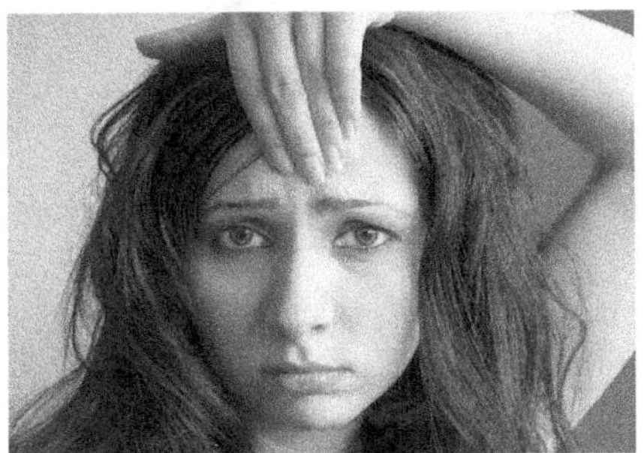

Remedies for Wrinkles

1. Drink at least 8 glasses of water per day and sleep adequately, to make skin tight and wrinkles free.
2. Vitamin A rich foods such as Carrot, Tomato, Cabbage (Patta gobi), Coriander (Dhania), Amaranth (Cholayi), Mango, Papaya, Orange, Milk, Butter can be taken, which helps to overcome wrinkles problem.
3. Regularly applying Cabbage paste with a spoon of Honey on the face and washing face after an hour tightens skin and wrinkle free.
4. Doing exercises like, taking water or air in the mouth and transferring it from one side to another several times, tightens face skin and wrinkle free.

5. Open your mouth as wide as possible and then close as tight as possible several times, this exercise helps to get wrinkle free face.

6. Regularly massaging face with Castor oil (Erand) or Coconut oil makes face wrinkle free.

7. Beat egg whites of two eggs and apply on the face and wash the face with cold water after half an hour which helps in reducing wrinkles on the face.

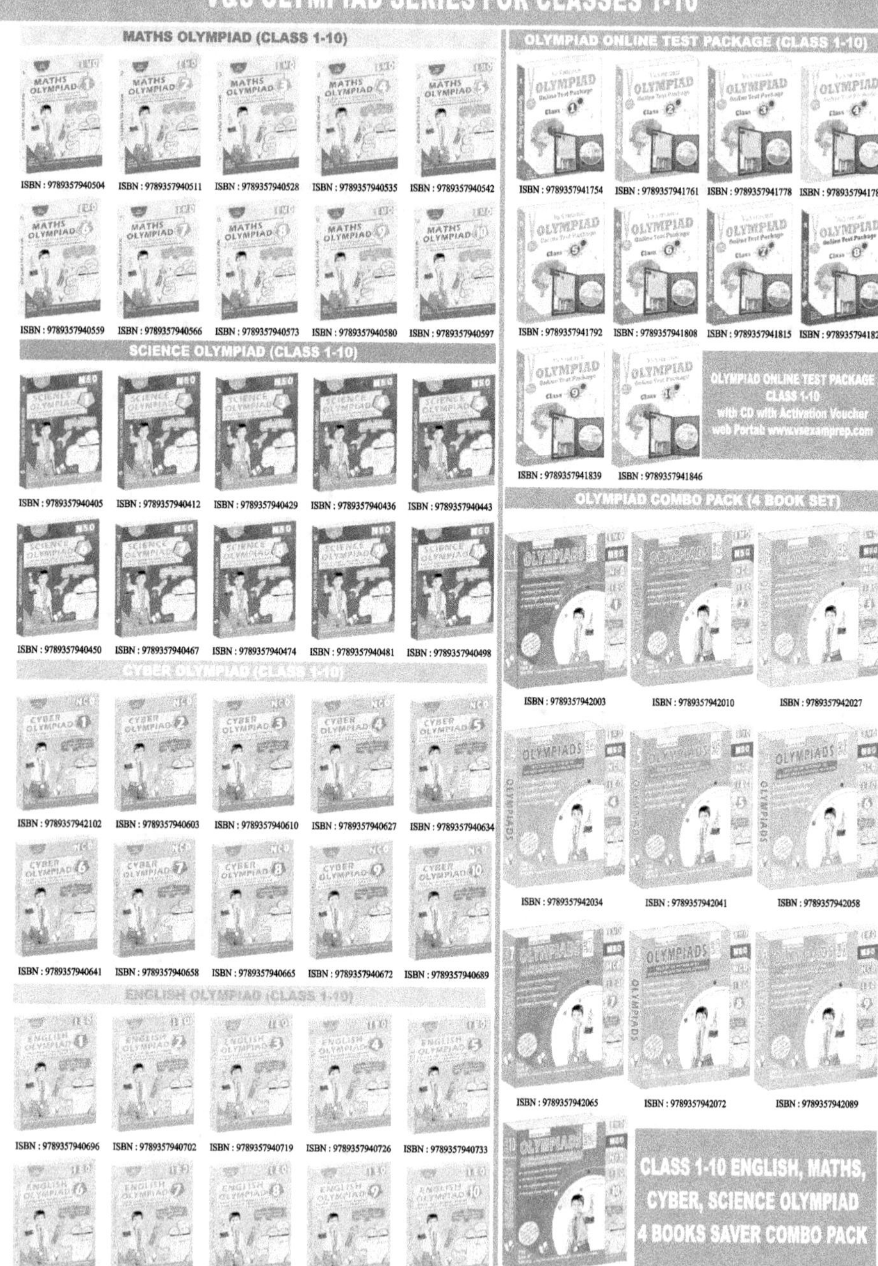

V&S OLYMPIAD SERIES FOR CLASSES 1-10

MATHS OLYMPIAD (CLASS 1-10)
ISBN : 9789357940504
ISBN : 9789357940511
ISBN : 9789357940528
ISBN : 9789357940535
ISBN : 9789357940542
ISBN : 9789357940559
ISBN : 9789357940566
ISBN : 9789357940573
ISBN : 9789357940580
ISBN : 9789357940597

SCIENCE OLYMPIAD (CLASS 1-10)
ISBN : 9789357940405
ISBN : 9789357940412
ISBN : 9789357940429
ISBN : 9789357940436
ISBN : 9789357940443
ISBN : 9789357940450
ISBN : 9789357940467
ISBN : 9789357940474
ISBN : 9789357940481
ISBN : 9789357940498

CYBER OLYMPIAD (CLASS 1-10)
ISBN : 9789357942102
ISBN : 9789357940603
ISBN : 9789357940610
ISBN : 9789357940627
ISBN : 9789357940634
ISBN : 9789357940641
ISBN : 9789357940658
ISBN : 9789357940665
ISBN : 9789357940672
ISBN : 9789357940689

ENGLISH OLYMPIAD (CLASS 1-10)
ISBN : 9789357940696
ISBN : 9789357940702
ISBN : 9789357940719
ISBN : 9789357940726
ISBN : 9789357940733
ISBN : 9789357940740
ISBN : 9789357940757
ISBN : 9789357940764
ISBN : 9789357940771
ISBN : 9789357940788

OLYMPIAD ONLINE TEST PACKAGE (CLASS 1-10)
ISBN : 9789357941754
ISBN : 9789357941761
ISBN : 9789357941778
ISBN : 9789357941785
ISBN : 9789357941792
ISBN : 9789357941808
ISBN : 9789357941815
ISBN : 9789357941822
ISBN : 9789357941839
ISBN : 9789357941846

OLYMPIAD ONLINE TEST PACKAGE
CLASS 1-10
with CD with Activation Voucher
web Portal: www.vsexamprep.com

OLYMPIAD COMBO PACK (4 BOOK SET)
ISBN : 9789357942003
ISBN : 9789357942010
ISBN : 9789357942027
ISBN : 9789357942034
ISBN : 9789357942041
ISBN : 9789357942058
ISBN : 9789357942065
ISBN : 9789357942072
ISBN : 9789357942089
ISBN : 9789357942096

CLASS 1-10 ENGLISH, MATHS,
CYBER, SCIENCE OLYMPIAD
4 BOOKS SAVER COMBO PACK

All Books Available on Flipkart, Amazon, Infibeam, Snapdeal, Shopclues • marketing@vspublishers.com

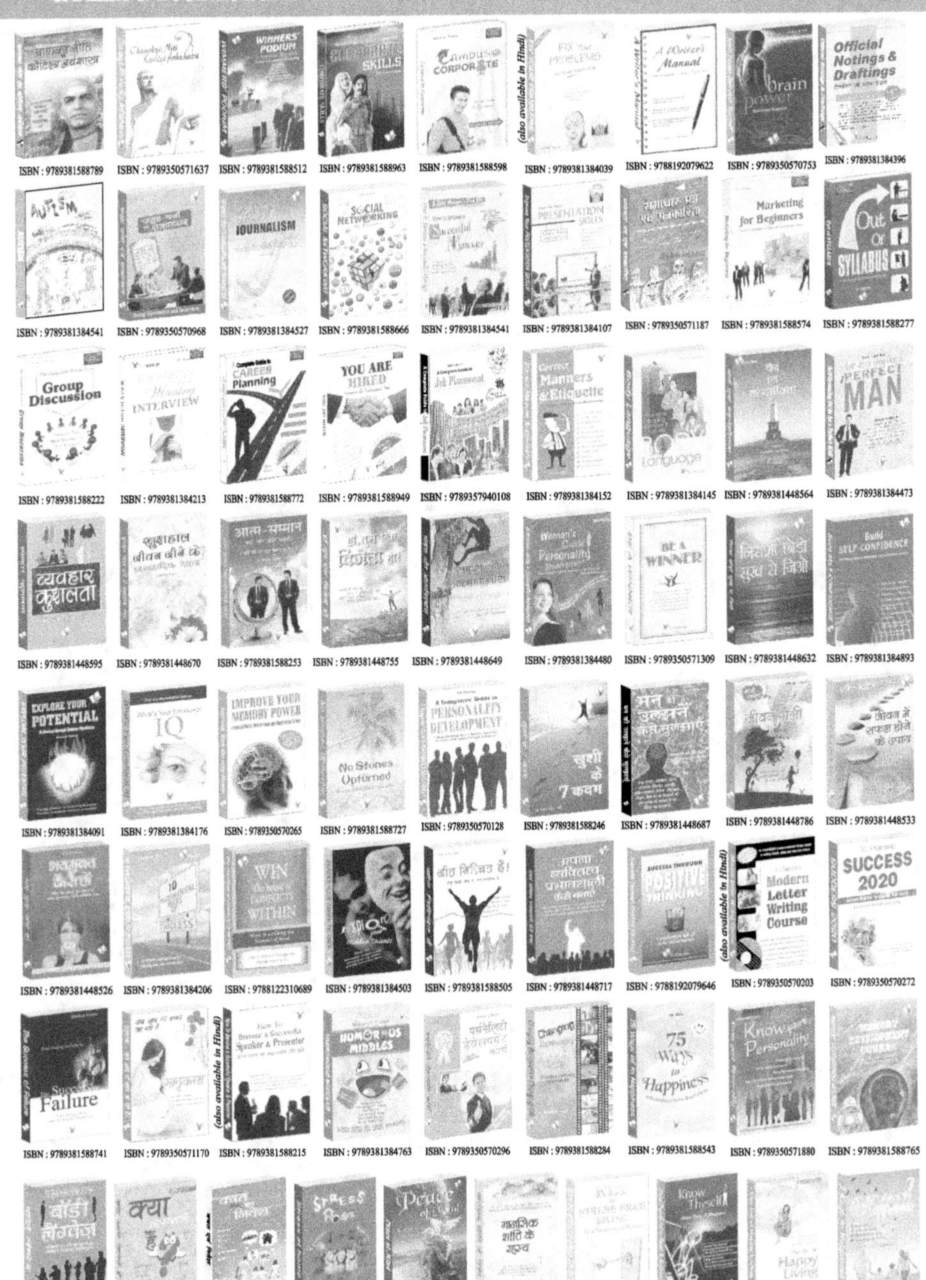

ISBN : 9789381588789   ISBN : 9789350571637   ISBN : 9789381588512   ISBN : 9789381588963   ISBN : 9789381588598   ISBN : 9789381384039   ISBN : 9788192079622   ISBN : 9789350570753   ISBN : 9789381384396

ISBN : 9789381384541   ISBN : 9789350570968   ISBN : 9789381384527   ISBN : 9789381588666   ISBN : 9789381384541   ISBN : 9789381384107   ISBN : 9789350571187   ISBN : 9789381588574   ISBN : 9789381588277

ISBN : 9789381588222   ISBN : 9789381384213   ISBN : 9789381588772   ISBN : 9789381588949   ISBN : 9789357940108   ISBN : 9789381384152   ISBN : 9789381384145   ISBN : 9789381448564   ISBN : 9789381384473

ISBN : 9789381448595   ISBN : 9789381448670   ISBN : 9789381588253   ISBN : 9789381448755   ISBN : 9789381448649   ISBN : 9789381384480   ISBN : 9789350571309   ISBN : 9789381448632   ISBN : 9789381384893

ISBN : 9789381384091   ISBN : 9789381384176   ISBN : 9789350570265   ISBN : 9789381588727   ISBN : 9789350570128   ISBN : 9789381588246   ISBN : 9789381448687   ISBN : 9789381448786   ISBN : 9789381448533

ISBN : 9789381448526   ISBN : 9789381384206   ISBN : 9788122310689   ISBN : 9789381384503   ISBN : 9789381588505   ISBN : 9789381448717   ISBN : 9788192079646   ISBN : 9789350570203   ISBN : 9789350570272

ISBN : 9789381588741   ISBN : 9789350571170   ISBN : 9789381588215   ISBN : 9789381384763   ISBN : 9789350570296   ISBN : 9789381588284   ISBN : 9789381588543   ISBN : 9789350571880   ISBN : 9789381588765

ISBN : 9789350570579   ISBN : 9789350571927   ISBN : 9789350571545   ISBN : 9789381384114   ISBN : 9789381384435   ISBN : 9789381448779   ISBN : 9789381448991   ISBN : 9789381384510   ISBN : 9789381384169   ISBN : 9789350570623